Managing Your Memory

PRACTICAL SOLUTIONS
FOR FORGETTING

Bill E. Beckwith, Ph.D.

Managing Your Memory:
Practical Solutions for Forgetting

Copyright © 2004 Bill E. Beckwith, Ph.D.

PUBLISHED BY
Memory Management
Post Office Box 07088
Fort Myers, FL 33919
INTERNET: www.memorymanagement.info
E-MAIL: info@memorymanagement.info

First Edition

ISBN 0-9748379-1-1
Library of Congress Control Number: 2004105725

PRODUCED BY
Boulder Bookworks, Boulder, Colorado
www.boulderbookworks.com

Printed in the United States of America

To my wife, Pamela,

for visions that nudged
and inspired me,
and for your love.

Acknowledgments

I gratefully acknowledge my mentor and friend Curt Sandman who provided the intellectual freedom from which I have grown more than he can know. I also wish to thank Cass Leoncini and Kim Waltman who read an earlier, very rough draft of this manuscript. Finally, my deep appreciation to Mary Anne Maier for her compassionately thorough editing and Alan Bernhard for guiding me through the many challenges of having my ideas become a real book.

Contents

Introduction

I am now in my late 50s, and this book has given me the opportunity to look back at my own experiences with memory. I have been interested in how memory works at least since I had to memorize a passage from *Macbeth* as a senior in high school. I also had to master my memory in order to efficiently study and learn during my years of undergraduate and graduate training.

As an educator (ranging from preschool to junior high, college, and graduate education) for 15 years, I helped others learn and remember. I have published many papers in professional journals on numerous aspects of learning and memory in humans and in animals. During the past 13 years in private practice as a memory specialist, I have created a comprehensive memory management center and consulted with hundreds of older people with inefficient or declining memories. At the same time, I have contended with the changes in efficiency of my own memory as I get older. My conclusion from these many years of experience with memory is that there are simply no shortcuts to a better memory.

It is clear to me that the memory skill that allows me to learn and retain new information and keeps me from being overly absentminded does not benefit from exercise, or "mental aerobics." I have learned many skills and a great deal of information during my life, but I have always had to put time and effort into this process. As I grow older I have to use more notes, rely on a more detailed calendar, and keep myself more organized. In short, I am aware that I have to manage my short-term and working memory as the brain systems that regulate these faculties become less efficient with each decade that I continue to live. Despite these changes I plan to be able to successfully enjoy my life and recall my experiences. If I practice what I preach (and I do not develop a disorder of memory), I will learn and grow, to paraphrase Carl Rogers, as long as I live.

This book is not an attempt to be encyclopedic in coverage; rather, I have tried to distill information that has been helpful to me in developing my professional appreciation of normal and abnormal memory as well as in understanding how to better use my own memory. This book was developed to be practical rather than academic. Therefore, I chose not to use a scholarly format of referencing ideas. The reference section at the end of the book contains many sources that I have found to be helpful in extending my grasp of learning and memory. The conclusions contained in this book represent my understanding of memory and its management and are based on my personal experience of trying to master information as I have progressed through my life as well as on my professional knowledge of memory.

I have worked with persons younger than I with memory loss as well as persons who, like me, are struggling with managing the normal changes in the efficiency of memory as we age. I have worked with people with memory loss resulting from neurological disorders (head injury, Alzheimer's disease, stroke) as well as medical disorders (kidney disease, heart disease, diabetes). In none of these contexts are there easy ways to a better memory. Although there are exercises and experiences that strengthen or reinforce memory, unfortunately there are no exercises that strengthen memory *abilities*.

But the strategies that reinforce and strengthen memory described in this book help support memory whether you are 10 or 90. These strategies are helpful for those facing the changes of aging as well as the challenges of illnesses that interfere with memory. The techniques described here involve spending more time and effort in deciding what is important to learn and track. These techniques require that you use your cleverness to manage information and to compensate for changes that range from aging to "having too much to remember."

This book is organized into three major sections. The first section consists of nine chapters that are meant to help you 1) better understand memory, and 2) develop and use specific techniques to more effectively learn and remember new information, remember what needs to be done when, and remember where to go and how to get there. The chapters in this section describe the concept of what memory is as well as factors that influence forgetting. These chapters also discuss the changes that can be expected during aging and the techniques that have been proven to help support learning and memory regardless of age.

The second section consists of two chapters, 10 and 11, describing disorders of memory and the concepts of Mild Cognitive Impairment, dementia, and Alzheimer's disease. They are the most technical chapters in the book. The third section, containing chapters 12 through 15, outlines issues related to managing controllable factors such as diet and exercise that may improve mental operations as we age and may slow down possible memory disorders. These chapters also contain information needed for planning ahead in case you have risk factors associated with the possible development of a memory disorder or if you already have mild changes in memory beyond those of normal aging.

We insure ourselves against certain financial contingencies. We create a road map for retirement. We should also get organized to protect ourselves against the inconveniences of aging and possible fading memory skills. If you have vulnerabilities for developing conditions such as Alzheimer's disease or stroke, planning ahead becomes critical for successful management of your future. Unfortunately, if you wait until you need the skills described in the first part of this book, you may no longer be able to learn them. That's why it's important to develop good memory "hygiene" so that you will have the skills before they are needed.

According to a recent *New York Times* article, many elders (a word I am increasingly finding distasteful but accurate for myself) fear developing Alzheimer's disease more than they fear their own death. This need not be the case as Alzheimer's disease progresses over the course of decades. The early phases of the disease produce annoyances and inconveniences. These inconveniences can be well managed by careful, advanced planning. It is never too early to plan ahead. Your memory is the best it will ever be. Now is the time to learn memory management skills *before* you need them. Design a plan to preserve your past for active conservation of your future. This book was written to assist you in this process.

The past is consumed in the present

and the present is living

only because it brings forth the future.

— JAMES JOYCE,
A Portrait of the Artist
as a Young Man

PART I

What Is Memory

and How Do You

Manage It?

CHAPTER ONE

How's Your Memory Hygiene?

I'm often asked, "How can I improve my memory?" or "Can I do exercises to improve my memory?" Whether you are simply anticipating or already experiencing the inefficiencies of memory that result from aging or are developing clinically significant memory loss, these are probably the wrong questions to ask. That's because memory is not a single skill. Instead, memory is a general term that covers several skills ranging from remembering our own name to remembering how to swim. None of us has a "good" or a "bad" memory. Some of us master new information quickly while others need to spend more time and effort at all points in our life to master new information. We all have various strengths and weaknesses for remembering different kinds of information or different kinds of skills. For example, I may have a good memory for dates but a poor memory for when to take medications. You may have a good memory for driving a car with an automatic transmission but a poor memory for driving a car with a manual transmission.

In other words, what we generally refer to as our memory is actually a complex set of skills and abilities with a pattern of personal strengths and weaknesses. I can remember my name, my birth date, and my siblings' names. I remember facts and concepts that I have learned during my education. I remember vacations that I have taken but often do not recall specific details such as what I did on which day. I remember odors (my wife's perfume), tastes (strawberry shortcake), feelings (sadness from deaths of persons or pets for whom I have cared). There are many avenues to remembering. Not all of my memories are in the form of words or concepts. I know and can recall much more than I can say. Memories have different ways of being organized and stored in the brain. Memories are structured and recalled in accordance with my personal views, my likes, and my dislikes. Furthermore, memory skills cannot be strengthened like a muscle. Repetition increases the strength of the memory but not the skill of forming or consolidating the memory in the first place. That is why memory skills must be managed. This book is designed to help you better manage your memory.

Before examining the definition of memory, consider the following questions about your own memory. The more often you answer "yes" to these questions, the better your memory "hygiene," or memory management skills. If you answer "no" to several of the questions, you have some work to do.

1. Do you use a timer or alarm to remind you to do something?

2. Do you ask someone else to remind you to do something or to help you remember?

3. Do you write things on a calendar? Do you include pleasurable activities? Do you include appointments? Do you include routines that you wish to build?

4. Do you have a "to do" list? Do you update it each day? Do you have more items on the "to do" list than you can possibly manage in a day?

5. When you are stumped about a word or a name, do you go through the alphabet one letter at a time to see if it brings to mind the word or name?

6. Do you say something out loud in order to remember it? Do you write it down to help you remember it?

7. Do you use routines to help you remember important things? Does everything have a place and is everything in its place?

8. Do you make lists to recall what to buy at the grocery store? Do you remember to take the list with you?

9. Do you mentally elaborate on something that you want to remember? Do you try to form associations? Do you try to conjure up an image, a story, a rhyme?

10. Do you put things that are important to remember in a prominent place to remind you to do something or to take something with you?

11. Do you repeat information to yourself at increasingly longer and longer intervals so that you will remember it? Do you plan practice opportunities to help keep important skills sharp or to develop new skills that you wish to acquire?

12. Do you take notes to help you remember? Do you organize your notes and keep them in a convenient (and routine) place for easy use? Do you update and review them often?

13. Do you use a tape recorder to help you remember?

CHAPTER TWO

Common Questions About Memory

The fundamental strategy for having a better memory is spending more time with information or skills and spending more time organizing/ practicing the information or skills. Experiences and skills we ponder or practice are much less prone to forgetting. If you are unfortunate enough to develop a disorder of memory (reviewed in chapters 10 and 11), developing the strategies described in the next seven chapters will help you to manage your life and memory for a much longer period of time. But everyone will experience decreased efficiency of memory as we age, so these strategies can help all of us to better manage our life and memory. The important thing to keep in mind is that if you wait until you "need" to master the techniques described below, it may be too late to learn to use them.

You will better remember information with which you spend more time and information that you anticipate. This chapter starts you on the process of building better memory hygiene by addressing questions and concerns that you might have about memory and at the same time introducing the basics of memory aids and memory management.

Are There Different Kinds of Memory?

Yes. I remember schedules and things I want and need to do (I am going on vacation in three weeks). I remember skills (how to ski, how to ride a bicycle). I remember routes (how to get home from work), names (my wife's name is Pamela, my cat's name is Pepper), and facts (the capital of North Dakota is Bismarck, the capital of South Dakota is pronounced "pier"). I remember movements (walking). I remember odors (the smell of fresh baked bread). I remember feelings (the happiness of seeing Pamela's smile). There are many different kinds of memory, and each may be organized by different memory systems and/or codes. The types of memory will be discussed in chapter 3.

What Changes Can I Expect in Memory Operations as I Age?

Senility is not a necessary consequence of aging. However, my memory will become less efficient as I grow older. I already see changes in the reliability and efficiency of my memory as I approach 60 compared to when I was in my early 50s. I am much more vulnerable to distraction (absentmindedness, blocking, and fading of memory) than I used to be. I need a much more detailed calendar. These changes will be discussed in chapter 4.

Is Forgetting Normal?

The answer is simple: Yes. We all forget, no matter how young or old we are. Memories generally fade with the passage of time. We recall the gist, the essence, but not the details. Very few of us have photographic memory, and those who do are usually quite young and may not find such detailed memories a blessing. Indeed, those with photographic memory are often frustrated by the detail they cannot help but recall. They may have difficulty seeing the forest for the trees, so to speak.

Forgetting is a normal part of memory and must be acknowledged and planned for. If you know the factors that increase the likelihood of forgetting, you can compensate for or work around them. Many, but not all, of us will most likely do better in challenging mental tasks that require memory and dependable attention in the mornings rather than in the evenings. This may reflect the effects of fatigue as the day wears on. We are more likely to recall information that is well organized, so we can better remember to pay the bills if bills are organized into folders and bill paying is marked on the calendar each month as an activity. We are more likely to recall a phone message if we repeat the message back to be sure we got it right. Factors that increase forgetting will be discussed in chapter 5.

Who Am I?

This is a basic question that needs to be addressed when deciding how to organize your memory. We all have skills, knowledge, and routines. What we pay attention to and remember depends upon who we are, our past experiences, our knowledge, and our needs. Our schemas and routines are the skeleton upon which we can structure memory skills.

For example, I shave first thing in the morning. That means that a note on the mirror that I use to shave will help me remember something that is important to do that day. Alternatively, placing a new medication that I need to take in the mornings next to my razor increases the likelihood that I will take it routinely. As another example, I have already developed adequate computer skills. This means that I can use computers to assist me in recalling what I need to do or to know. When I give seminars, I use a series of slides from my computer to provide the blueprint for the issues that I want to remember to discuss. Additionally, the slides help my audience to recall many of the major points that I will make because they see as well as hear the information that I have presented. Long-term memory is discussed in chapter 7.

What Is Abnormal Forgetting?

Abnormal forgetting is being more forgetful than my peers. In other words, if I am 58 years old, I would be abnormally forgetful if on a difficult memory test I recalled much less information than other 58-year-olds who have taken the same memory test. As an extreme example, consider that it is okay to occasionally forget where you parked your car. However, it is not okay to forget that you have a car. Abnormal forgetting is not the same thing as having "no" memory. People with abnormal forgetting may recall many things very well, but they have certain memory skills that are poor. Usually abnormal forgetting involves failure to adequately learn new things or adjust to change. Abnormal forgetting also usually refers to forgetting what you have to do (forgetting to take a new medication, forgetting appointments). Abnormal forgetting will be discussed in chapters 10 and 11.

What Kinds of Skills Should Be Evaluated during Memory Testing?

During a formal memory evaluation, information needs to be obtained not only from the person who has memory concerns but also from a knowledgeable family member or friend, if possible. The ability to learn new information should be evaluated with a challenging memory test. This memory test must examine the ability to recall newly learned information immediately as well as after a delay. It should also examine the ability to recognize newly learned information since some who have difficulty recalling the information may do well in recognizing it and will probably do better with external memory aids.

The evaluation should also obtain a careful history to learn who the person is (education, work skills, leisure skills) and to obtain information on the unfolding of the problems. This history also helps assess long-term memory skills. Other mental skills should also be queried such as language construction, problem solving, and executive skills (planning, judgment, intelligence). A clear understanding of the current state of these skills allows the development of a management plan that uses strengths to shore up weaknesses (if my writing is unintelligible, I should not write notes for myself).

Memory evaluations are complex and take time. If the memory test is easy, it is probably not useful. The most important aspect of the evaluation is the review and explanation of findings as this allows the person with concerns to develop a strategic plan. The findings should be reviewed in detail as they pertain to everyday skills as well as anticipated future changes. Evaluations are discussed in chapters 10 and 11.

What Are the Goals of Memory Management?

First, you must ask yourself, "Which kind of memory do I want to improve?" The answer then becomes simpler as the techniques that improve one kind of memory (how to ski) differ from those used to improve another kind of memory (tracking when to take the cake out of the oven). Memory can be improved by better management of existing memory capabilities and development of new memory know-how. Plan ahead. Learn skills before you need them. I need to plan ahead for getting older not only by anticipating retirement but also by designing strategies for dealing with changes in my physical and mental skills so that I can continue to enjoy my life and minimize my frustrations.

The major rules of memory management are easy: 1) Spend more time. 2) Organize, review, and associate. 3) Use routines. 4) Use external memory aids. 5) Minimize or plan for factors that contribute to forgetting. General rules for managing memory will be discussed in chapter 8.

What Techniques and Aids Can Be Successful for Managing Memory?

There are specific techniques that allow you to become more efficient at learning and recalling new as well as old information. These are techniques that use assistive strategies. They include using such external aids as timers, calendars, computers, and even other people. These techniques are described in chapter 9.

CHAPTER THREE

What Is Memory, Anyway?

I often have clients who come to me saying that they are concerned that there is something wrong with their memory. However, as I ask them questions about their birthday, the name of the high school from which they graduated, or their address and phone number, they provide the correct information. Furthermore, they are well groomed and dressed, suggesting that they recall how to care for themselves. They look well fed and fit, suggesting that they remember to eat and exercise. They are on time for their appointments, suggesting they have recalled when they are to meet with me. They have also found their way to my office, suggesting that they have adequate route-finding memory. They interact in socially appropriate ways, suggesting they recall social conventions. They can still swim if they ever learned in the first place. They recognize familiar persons, suggesting they have memory for faces. Still they report that they are concerned about how their memory is working. They fear that their memory is failing.

It seems that many of us have a sense that memory is an overall capacity or ability and that our "memory" is good or bad. Hence, we speak of fear of "losing our memory." However, there are a multitude of memory systems in the brain, and each has unique properties of operation. Furthermore, most of us have good memory in some areas (spelling) and poor in others (route finding). We have memory for language, movement, and music. We remember the multiplication tables, our family, and the locations of many familiar places. We recall our personal history and have memory of self. We have knowledge of skills such as touch typing or riding a bicycle. We recall sounds, sights, tastes, and odors. We also have memories of emotions. We remember when to take medications and when the trash will be collected. Memory is clearly not a general skill. Rather, memory is a concept that indicates many skills.

Anterograde Amnesia: The Case of H.M.

When people complain of "losing" their memory, they usually mean their "short-term memory." This is the memory system that allows us to learn new information. Aging as well as disorders of memory often produce failures of short-term and working memory (discussed later). The most well-known and thoroughly studied clinical case of short-term memory failure is that of H.M. H.M. grappled with epileptic seizures from childhood. In 1953, at the age of 27, H.M. was the first and only human known to have a brain structure, the hippocampus, removed from both sides of his brain by a neurosurgeon, William Scoville. This structure rests beneath the temporal lobes of the cerebral cortex.

The surgery was a success in that it reduced the severity of H.M.'s seizures. However, it created a new and unexpected problem, causing time to simply stop for H.M. After the surgery, he was unable to learn new facts. For example, he could

not learn the names of new presidents after 1951. Many
researchers and clinicians have met and spent considerable time
with H.M. over the past 50 years, but he always greeted even
those who worked with him over long periods as new to his life.
He recalled people from before the surgery but not new people.
He also could not learn new routes, such as how to get to and
from his room. In addition, he lost about two years of past or
remote memory as a result of the surgery. As far as he was concerned he was, and remains, a 25-year-old man. Although there
were things that he could learn after the surgery, such as how to
trace figures while looking at them in a mirror, he did not know
that he knew them. He has reported that he has the constant
feeling that he is "awakening from a dream." H.M. lost a critical
skill of memory (storing new information) but did not lose
reality.

On a general level, we would say that H.M. had lost his
memory. However, he did not have a total loss of memory. He
still knew who he was and how to care for himself. He still
knew the past facts of his life, could learn new skills (although
he did not know that he knew them), and had the stores of
knowledge that he had before the surgery. This memory disorder, surgically produced in H.M.'s case, is known as *anterograde
amnesia*. It is the type of memory loss that most of us refer to
when we say that someone has lost his or her memory, though
H.M.'s case is much more severe. Most clients with memory loss
whom I have seen and assessed have a mild form of anterograde
memory loss. In Alzheimer's disease, and in what we will later
discuss as Mild Cognitive Impairment, the memory loss is also
that of short-term memory, or anterograde amnesia. In this most
common type of memory loss, the ability to learn new information is impaired. It usually appears to be a disorder involving
changes in the hippocampus but may also be found with damage to other brain structures in the thalamus and limbic system.

What Is Memory?

According to *Merriam-Webster's Collegiate Dictionary* (10th edition, 1998), memory is "the power or process of reproducing or recalling what has been learned and retained." Alternatively, memory is "the store of things learned and retained from an organism's activity or experience as evidenced by modification of structure or behavior or by recall and recognition." Note that memory is an enduring change in "structure" or "behavior" that results from "experience" or "learning," which implies changes in function and structure of the brain. In other words, memory is the capacity to learn and to retain new information, to recall the information or skill when needed, and to recognize instances of familiarity when we are exposed to parts of information or experience in the future.

In order to better understand the complexity of memory, let's explore some major aspects of our memory. This understanding will help us later to disentangle changes in memory that result from normal aging as well as those that occur as a result of memory disorders. The major types of memory are *sensory, primary, working, short-term, long-term, procedural, prospective,* and *emotional memory*. Although this discussion is not exhaustive, it will help put memory in a larger context and show how some memory skills are retained even in those with memory disorders. It is the retained skills that need to be exploited to manage memory loss as well as to allow a continuing sense of competence and joy.

Sensory Memory

Sensory memory is a temporary impression left on the sense organs after perception. It is sort of like an after-image. Sensory memory is very transient and is quickly lost. It is a momentary total representation of a stimulus, such as a word or image heard or seen, that is rich in details: a face observed, sound heard, a touch felt. These memories endure for less than a second and are passive. Sensory memory works in all of us unless we lose a sense such as hearing or suffer certain kinds of brain injury such as a stroke. Managing sensory memory requires that we do what we can to keep our senses as sharp as possible to assist memory processes later in the chain. The most obvious way to manage sensory memory is to wear hearing aids or eye corrections. While our sensory memory can become less efficient, this is not the type of memory that leads people to say they have problems with their memory.

Primary Memory

Primary memory is a second form of temporary memory. Primary memory is the memory system that we use to look up and dial a phone number that we will no longer need. It holds about seven (plus or minus two) pieces of information that will remain available as long as rehearsal (repeating the information in your mind) occurs.

Information is lost through interference as new information displaces the old. Hence, the phone number called just once is lost as you begin your conversation. Distraction also interferes with primary memory. If I go into another room for something and am distracted (by my wife talking to me, perhaps, or an intrusive thought popping into my head), I may forget what I went into the room to do or to get. Primary memory lasts for seconds (up to about a minute) unless we actively rehearse the information without distraction. It can hold only a limited amount of information, about the length of a phone number. While our primary memory can become less efficient, this is also not the kind of memory that commonly leads people to say they have problems with memory.

Working Memory

Working memory is a third type of temporary memory system. Working memory and primary memory are not distinct systems, but they do somewhat different tasks. One way to understand these functions of memory is to think of primary memory as a passive system to hold information and working memory as an active system to manipulate the information. If primary memory allows me to hold seven items, working memory allows me to manipulate them. One way to test your working memory is to try repeating a phone number you know backwards.

Working memory allows me to decipher information and to track multiple things at the same time. For example, working memory allows me to listen to a lecture while taking notes. It allows me to interpret the meaning of the words and concepts the speaker is using. Working memory also allows me to track what I have to do and when I have to do it. In fact, working memory is critical to our understanding of language and our keeping to our plans. It is highly influenced by attention and interference. Declines in working memory rather than primary memory are something we must all compensate for as we age. Our working memory is related to yet another temporary memory function that is named prospective memory.

Prospective Memory

We must all track events (plans with visitors, appointments and engagements, the need to return someone's call) and time (how long the cake needs to bake, when we need to go to an appointment or engagement, when we need to take medications). This is the function of prospective memory, which is another temporary memory system that is probably connected to working memory as it requires sharing our attention over time. This is another system that is subject to growing less efficient as we age. Prospective memory allows us to monitor and interact with our future whereas other memory functions/systems that we have discussed so far connect us to the past.

Short-Term Memory

Short-term memory is another relatively temporary memory system. Short-term memory holds information that endures for minutes to hours to days. Obviously, short-term memory constantly interacts with sensory, primary, working, and prospective memory. It is the harmony of these systems that allows us to function smoothly most of the time in our everyday life.

Short-term memory adds the function of allowing us to accumulate new information and knowledge. This is the system by which we learn new information, behaviors, and skills. Short-term memory allows me to learn new names and facts and to build my store of knowledge. It also allows me to link the past, present, and future. H.M.'s surgery produced severe deficits in his short-term memory, which we call severe anterograde amnesia. Short-term memory becomes less proficient with aging and is susceptible to many kinds of injuries and illnesses. Yet short-term memory allows the accumulation of information and skills that builds long-term memory.

Long-Term Memory

Long-term memory is a more or less permanent memory. It is based on information being stored by the brain that is available for use at later times. It is our personal history, our store of knowledge, our enduring self, and our persisting skills. Long-term memory changes as a result of experience. Mental exercises and stimulation, referred to by some as "memory aerobics," are believed by some to protect memory and to ward off Alzheimer's disease. But mental exercises have been shown to strengthen long-term memory, not short-term, working, primary, sensory, or prospective memory. Doing crossword puzzles builds skills of long-term memory but does not strengthen or improve short-term memory ability or efficiency. Long-term memory (despite its many foibles) works quite well even in many with disorders of memory. Thus long-term memory is the strength that we can build on if we detect memory disorders in their very early stages.

There are numerous functions that the memory systems described so far carry out to make our life smooth and allow us to learn and to interact with our world. So far we have focused on systems that allow information and skills to enter into our repertoire of knowledge, behaviors, and self. Another important distinction that is helpful in understanding how memory works is the distinction between declarative and procedural memory. Declarative memory is based on language use. It is episodic (recalling the date) or semantic (recalling a fact or piece of personal information from our knowledge system). Declarative memory allows us to know that we know; it is knowing "that." Procedural memory represents memory that allows us to do; it permits us to know "how."

Procedural Memory

Procedural memory is the memory of skills and procedures. We recall how to walk, dress, chew, and swallow. We recall how to ride bicycles, how to swim, or how to touch type. These are not activities that we have to think about doing. Procedural memories unfold without thought. They are automatic. Indeed, if we try to think about the elements involved in a skill such as walking, we interfere with the process and may stumble or get our legs crossed up. We are not used to thinking in order to walk; we just do it.

Procedural memories are developed and strengthened by repetition and practice. As I age, it takes me more time to build procedural memories. For example, those who learn to ski when they are young are generally much better skiers than those who learn when they are adults. It is much easier to learn languages when we are young than when we are adults because the process of learning languages seems to be different for children, more automatic, while it is more rote for adults. I have often marveled at the computer skills of those growing up with computers compared to me learning to use a computer as an adult. Procedural memory is another strength, along with long-term memory, upon which we can build even if we develop memory loss.

Emotional Memory

The final type of memory that I would like to discuss is emotional memory. Emotional memory is the store of feelings and reactions that we have to situations and people. Emotional memory may be positive (feelings of love toward my wife, joy of accomplishment) or may be negative (waves of sorrow during grieving, fear and apprehension when the plane in which I am flying encounters turbulence). Emotional memory can be triggered by cues, incidents, or thoughts. For example, if you have speech anxiety, standing (or merely thinking about standing) in front of an audience may make you very anxious and elicit the desire to run away or to avoid giving speeches. Emotional memory, like long-term memory, persists. We often think of memory as neutral. However, memory and behavior are strongly influenced by emotions. Managing memory may include managing emotions. We shall discuss this topic further in chapter 14.

Although there are other important complications and nuances of memory that have not been addressed, I hope this discussion has helped to clarify some important distinctions and functions of memory. As we age, there are changes in our memory. These changes do not reduce our ability to enjoy life, to learn new information, or to monitor what we have to do. However, the growing inefficiency of short-term and working memory as we age causes us amusement (we develop "old-timer's" disease) and annoyances. The next step in appreciating the complexity of memory is to understand how the efficiency of our mental operations changes as we age.

CHAPTER FOUR

Normal Changes in Efficiency of Memory as We Age

As I look into the mirror each morning, I am aware that I have changed. I don't look like I did when I was 30. These changes are obvious. My hair is gray; my hairline is receding. I have more wrinkles. My skin has markings and blemishes that I did not have when I was younger. I don't always like these changes, but I can see them. They are obvious.

Consider how H.M. must feel when he looks into a mirror with the memory of a 25-year-old man and sees the image of a 77-year-old man.

What are not so obvious are the changes that have occurred in my internal organs. My bones have become less dense. My muscle strength and endurance have declined. My liver, kidneys, and heart have changed. All these bodily organs will continue to become less efficient as I age.

My brain will also change as I age. It will shrink. In fact, we have the largest number of cells that we will ever have in our brain by the age of two. The normal brain of a male at age 20 weights about 1400 grams (three pounds). By the ninth decade of life, the normal male brain will shrink to about 90-100 grams.

It will have some very tiny strokes and "blemishes." Indeed, it is very common to see brain imaging reports with descriptors such as "age associated" or "age consistent" atrophy or small vessel disease. I will develop some plaques and tangles in my brain (the pathology believed to underlie Alzheimer's disease). These changes will cause my cognitive skills (learning, perceiving, attending, problem solving) to become less efficient but will not necessarily lead me to develop dementia or senility as I age, even if I live into my 100s.

Memory loss and mental disability are not a necessary outcome of aging. Many of us will retain good memory and mental skills throughout our life span. Indeed, aging is not the antitheses of personal growth and creativity as some suggest. Our knowledge and vocabulary will increase as we age. And our fixed skills will remain intact (I recently had a mathematician client who is moderately demented quickly and accurately repeat back 10 digits – backwards!). Rather, as we age we experience a decline in working memory and capacity which will make us process information, solve problems, and think more slowly. This, in turn, will slow the speed at which we can acquire new information as well as reduce the amount of information that we can manage at any one time. We will also have more trouble directing our attention away from irrelevant information. For example, we may no longer be able to read while the radio is playing in the background.

These are the general inefficiencies that accompany aging. Knowing and planning for these changes allow you to manage your memory better no matter how old you are. Often these changes are subtle. The talents of a 20- or 30-year-old in the workplace are different from those of a 60- or 70-year-old in the same workplace. Given normal aging, the former will excel in tasks that require short-term and working memory while the latter will excel in tasks that require synthesis and experience.

It is important to plan for the following changes that will

occur as you age and put in place methods to compensate well before you need them.

Aging Produces Greater Difficulty in Dividing Attention

I have already noticed this in myself. I can no longer read in a noisy environment. I find that I must have a quiet place to absorb what I am reading. If I have background music while I work or read, the music must not contain words. I can no longer have the television on while I read anything that requires concentration. I have difficulty following a conversation if there is a second conversation going on in the background. I lose my place in conversation more often now than I used to. I need a more detailed calendar to track what I must do. It's a mistake for me to read my e-mail while I am on the phone. If I am asked to take a new or a second medication, I often have trouble consistently recalling that I need to do so.

Aging Requires You to Spend More Time and Effort in New Learning

I find this especially annoying when I am trying to learn a new name. I have always had a poor memory for names, but now I find that I have to see a new acquaintance multiple times before I can recall his or her name. Fortunately, I do much better with faces, and people are forgiving about my repeatedly having to ask for their name. If I am learning new information, I have found that taking notes and reviewing my notes helps even more than it did in the past. I have to travel new routes a few times to get them down well, especially when I travel to new places. The changes are quite subtle, but clearly I spend more time with learning new things than I feel I did in the past.

Aging Lengthens the Time Required to Bring a Piece of Information or a Word to Mind

I think more slowly as I age. My wife and I are movie buffs. We often discuss movies that we have seen. I find that I take longer to recall the names of movies that I have seen in the past or the names of actors that I have enjoyed watching than I used to. Sometimes I remember the name of the movie the day after I originally tried to recall it.

I also find this in conversations when I must choose an alternate word for the one I really want but can't remember. The words or concepts I want often come to me after the conversation has turned elsewhere. I am especially likely to block proper names and nouns. Despite the fact that my vocabulary will continue to grow at least into my 70s, my speed of finding words will decline for each decade I continue to live. Many confuse the slowness of word finding with loss of memory. Often people I know who are older than 70 are aware of these changes and find them very frustrating. These changes can be one of the signs of failing memory, but often they are not.

Aging Produces More Unintended Words

Sometimes I find myself using substitute or wrong words, especially nouns, for the concepts that I want. I recently was listening to a news broadcast in which a well-known and experienced anchor used the wrong word in a story and was apparently unaware he had even made this substitution. Seeing him made me feel a whole lot better when I recently was making a point about memory in a lecture and said "spring" when I meant to say "fall" as the current season. I am sure that I have used wrong words that neither I nor my audience even noticed.

CHAPTER FIVE

Things That Increase Forgetting

Although some theories have suggested that we remember everything we encounter in life, either consciously or unconsciously, forgetting is actually a natural part of memory. Even long-term memory is subject to change and forgetting. Memory is not fixed but rather is a flexible and variable store of fragments (making up the gist, or essence) that are subject to change. Hence the controversy over the reliability of eye-witness recall and testimony. Indeed, most of us would probably say that we would like to easily recall anything we wish without the frustration of forgetting. However, the process of forgetting may be as important to mental functions as is the process of remembering since forgetting helps us to think more creatively and synthesize information.

For example, the story of S. is a classical case study by the Russian psychologist A.R. Luria of a person who had too good a memory. S. was a reporter for a newspaper in Moscow. It is reported that S. was once reprimanded by his editor for not taking notes during a meeting. However, S. was able to recite back to his boss the precise contents of the meeting despite not taking notes. In several years of testing, Dr. Luria could not find any limits to S.'s capacity to recall detail. S. did not forget even long tables of seemingly random numbers. He could repeat the contents of such tables within an hour or years later and could reproduce the tables forwards or backwards from memory. S. did not forget with either distraction or time. Yet despite this remarkable ability, S. was generally disorganized and without direction. His ability to recall everything came at the price of not being able to form general impressions or draw meaning from events. Thus S.'s case demonstrates that rather than a blessing, the ability not to forget appears to be a curse. Either extreme, remembering too much or remembering too little, presents limitations that have to be managed. S. in fact spent a great deal of time and effort trying to forget!

Most of us have memories that function at a level somewhere between those of H.M. and S. This means that most of us must deal with forgetting and the imperfections of memory. Daniel Schacter has suggested that memory has "seven sins," which serve well to illustrate the complexity of memory and forgetting. The seven sins of memory as defined by Schacter are transience, absentmindedness, blocking, misattribution, suggestibility, bias, and persistence. The first three of these sins, or what we might call simple memory flaws, are the ones that most of us increasingly struggle with on a conscious level in everyday life, and problems with them increase as we age.

Transience, the first memory sin, or flaw, refers to the fading of memory over time. Details of what we learn tend to fade in favor of central themes and gist. Transience is a function of the properties of working and short-term memory and is made worse by time and interference. The more we ponder or practice an experience, skill, or piece of information, the more resistant it becomes to transience. Absentmindedness results from dividing our attention and is driven by the properties of primary, working, and prospective memory. We spend so much of our time on autopilot in order to carry out routines that we often forget what we are told or what we have to do. Distinctive cues (external memory aids that we will discuss later) reduce absentmindedness. Blocking refers to the evasive name or word that will not come to mind when we want it. This is demonstrated by the tip-of-the-tongue experience and increases as we age. The best solutions to this frustration are time (if you wait the word or name may come to you) or searching the alphabet for the first letter of the name or word you want.

The fourth memory flaw is misattribution, which refers to our tendency to forget the source of a given memory. Misattribution also increases as we age. How many of the thoughts that we have are truly original? There are numerous examples of lawsuits where someone has written as their own someone else's thoughts (a sin I hope I have been able to avoid here). As our memories age, we tend to forget their origin. Plagiarism is often not intentional but rather results from forgetting the source of our thoughts or ideas and may increase as a particular memory ages. Another infrequent example of misattribution is the experience of deja vu. This experience is founded on the fact that we often remember as an experience of familiarity rather than as detail. Misattribution allows the con artist to engage in the "Where's the check?" scam. Here a contact is made, perhaps a phone call to gather information, to establish a sense of familiarity. After a short time, the person called forgets the details but experiences a sense of familiarity when the con artist calls back, allowing the con artist to make a false claim, such as, "Our records indicate that you paid $160, leaving a balance of only $60. Please make out a check for $60 to clear the balance."

Suggestibility refers to a process similar to misattribution but is not generally a problem encountered in everyday life. Rather, suggestibility is more likely to occur in legal and clinical contexts. Suggestibility creates complications in the legal processes of line-up identification, witness interrogation, and false confessions. Suggestibility also underlies many of the experiences that occur under hypnosis and the "false memory syndrome" where, for example, one recovers "lost" memories of trauma. Yet another memory flaw, bias, refers to our tendency to reconstruct our memory to fit with our own biases, needs, and views of the world. For example, we tend to view the past as consistent with the present. If we are depressed, we tend to recall our failures rather than our successes. If we buy a car that is too expensive, we immediately engage in rationalizations to justify our spending more than we can afford. If we smoke, we create elaborate justifications of our behavior. Hindsight, egocentricity, and stereotypes drive bias in our memories. This tendency to reconstruct memory to fit with our biases is the price we pay for being able to generalize.

Finally, persistence is the opposite of transience. Persistence is often driven by disappointment, failure, or trauma. Persistence occurs when we have a tune that we cannot get out of our head, or when we fall in love and cannot (and do not want to) get the person of our affections out of our head. Persistence produces the symptoms of grief and rumination. It underlies waking in the middle of the night to recall what we forgot to do (absentmindedness) earlier that day. Persistence is the usual outcome of trauma such as being robbed, assaulted, or abused. Persistence is driven by strong emotions that make certain experiences stand out from the background of life. These emotions take us immediately out of autopilot. The best treatment for persistence is disclosure and repetition of the feeling. The bereaved continue to repeatedly experience waves of sadness until acute pain subsides over a period of months to years.

Now that we better understand the naturalness and complexity of forgetting and memory distortion, we are ready to discuss how to manage forgetting. I hope I have convinced you that your memory will never be perfect. Still, there are many controllable factors that influence forgetting. Expecting and managing factors that we know increase the odds of forgetting is another aspect of good memory hygiene.

Not Paying Attention

If I don't pay attention in the first place, I will forget. Unlike S., I took notes in classes to help me recall what was said. However, taking notes made it harder to follow complex points and to keep up with lecturers who presented information too fast. It was sometimes challenging to take notes and to listen carefully at the same time, but not taking notes increased the effect of transience. Another situation that increases forgetting is having someone next to you say something as someone is lecturing. The well-meaning friend makes it harder to pay attention to the speaker. Also, being ill, daydreaming, taking medications or drugs, or being tired can interfere with attention. Pulling an "all-nighter" was never conducive to studying or listening to lectures when I was younger, and it would be even more detrimental to my remembering now. Another practical example of not attending well is couples who often talk to each other while in different rooms. Such couples might find it more helpful for their attention and thus their memory to go to the same room, turn off the TV, and make eye contact with the person to whom they are speaking. This improves the ability of each party to better attend to the communication. We can also improve our ability to pay attention by getting enough rest and doing more mentally demanding activities when we are most alert. Strategies such as these can help attention and thereby improve memory as aging reduces efficiency of processes such as attending to multiple tasks at the same time.

Distraction

I get distracted by thinking of things that I have to do. As I am talking with someone, I sometimes lose my train of thought (blocking) as I try to construct my arguments or as I am thinking of what I am going to say rather than listening to what the other person is saying. Movement that I catch with the corner of my eye may distract my attention and cause me to lose track of what I am doing or where I am going. The radio or television in the background may distract me from reading. Background conversations in a restaurant sometimes make it hard for me to listen to the person sitting next to me.

Distraction increases forgetting. Recall that primary, working, and short-term memory are subject to interference and distraction. Distractions can range from a phone ringing, a knock at the door, or a television show in the background to daydreaming or intrusive thoughts. Distraction can also be the result of using too many notes as reminders. The multiple notes fight each other for attention. Clutter can distract. Working in a clean and organized environment usually improves mental efficiency. Sometimes distraction and background noise produce stress. My wife and I recently stayed in a lake cabin without television or telephones. We also forgot the charger for the cell phone, so it quit working. It was such a treat, and a great stress reducer, to have the world of distractions minimized for a time.

Stress

Stress is another enemy of good memory. I recall the first time I tried to lecture. I had worked very hard writing out the lecture in detail. I spent considerable time practicing and rehearsing the material so I could become comfortable with it. However, when I actually had to present the lecture to a live audience, I felt my mind go blank, and I lost my place often in the written version of the lecture. As if this weren't enough, I completely lost my composure when someone asked a question.

To this day, I don't know how or why I persisted to finally master this terrible anxiety and become a lecturer. Since then, I have learned how to organize information better, manage my feelings, and use stress as my ally rather than my adversary. However, it is interesting how well I recall the emotions and feelings from those early experiences lecturing (persistence) despite the fact that I don't recall the specific information. Managing emotions and stress can contribute to more efficient memory and will be discussed in chapter 14.

Depression

Depression also distorts memory (bias) and may induce forgetting. In the extreme case, depression makes an individual so inner-focused on feelings of despair that the person cannot manage pertinent information from his or her surroundings. Furthermore, depression does not allow a person to focus on what is positive but rather causes the depressed person to focus on all that is wrong and all of his or her failings. There is a complex relationship between depression and forgetting.

Many professionals still believe that it is important to differentiate depression from dementia. Depression is seen as a "treatable" cause of dementia for some. The term "pseudodementia" was coined to emphasize this distinction. Self reports of memory loss by those who are depressed have been viewed by these professionals as examples of depressed persons' tendency to report that their traits, including memory, are bad. These professionals hypothesized that if the depression were successfully treated, the memory loss would go away. Unfortunately, this does not seem to be the case. We now know that while there may be some whose memory loss is explained by depression, it is much more likely that persons who demonstrate memory loss and depression as they get older will show future mental decline. These people need to manage their memory early. This will be discussed in chapter 11.

Loss and Grief

Loss and grief interfere with memory. One protective mechanism that we have to manage extreme psychic pain is to become "numb." We seem to act without awareness. This may be a good defense to help us manage extreme emotions, but it is very destructive to good memory operations.

The bereaved often do unusual things without apparent thinking and make poor decisions during the early stages of bereavement. Once they have "recovered" from the loss, they are amazed when others reflect on their actions and behaviors. Hence the suggestion that one make no major decisions during the first year of bereavement. It is also interesting how the image of the deceased appears to change during the course of grief. It seems that part of the process of grieving is the reconstruction of the memory of the deceased. This process is the opposite of that of the person who is depressed and focuses solely on negative traits and experiences. Rather, the bereaved person seems to "forget" the negative and remember the positive (bias). Thus the early stages of bereavement are not usually a time to do productive intellectual or mental work.

Lack of Organization

A lack of organization in daily life is a major pitfall for maintaining good memory. I make stacks of things that I feel I need to remember to do. I have multiple stacks. Often, I have been embarrassed to find a note buried under one of my stacks reminding me to make a phone call or respond to correspondence that I should have taken care of months before. Too many notes in too many places fight with each other for attention and thereby increase forgetting. Once I had to take a medication twice a day, once in the morning and once in the evening. I tied the morning medication to shaving and this worked very well. However, rather than organizing a routine for taking the evening medication, I "tried" to remember to take it sometime before I went to bed. Needless to say, I forgot that medication often and had to devise a more organized plan.

The solution to this weakness is to organize and "de-clutter." If you have not attended to an item in a stack during the first month, you will probably not get to it and in fact have likely already forgotten it. As part of your reorganization, make priorities and use distinctive cues and routines to combat prospective memory failures.

Illness

We're never at our best when we're ill or in pain. If I have a fever or a gastrointestinal bug, I will have more trouble with my memory. If I suffer from sleep apnea, so will my memory. Don't count on your memory during times of illness or injury. The illness and/or the medications to treat the problem may increase forgetting (contribute to transience). Don't do mentally demanding things when you are ill. Your memory will recover once you have recovered.

Medications

There are many medications that make our memory less efficient and few that make it better. For example, medications such as Valium, Klonopin, Ativan, or Xanax are good at inducing relaxation and reducing anxiety. However, they also cause subtle impairment in working and short-term memory. In other words, they can increase forgetting. Some antidepressant and pain medications also induce forgetting, as do over-the-counter sleep and allergy medications. There are abundant medications that can be included on this list of memory inhibitors.

The effects of medications on mental operations are complicated by the fact that some of us are more susceptible to deleterious influences of medications than are others. Forgetting is tied to dosage, timing, and frequency of taking a medication. Additionally, the effects of medications are often magnified during the process of aging. As we age there are alterations in the efficiency of our liver, lungs, cardiovascular system, gastrointestinal system, and kidneys. These changes influence the absorption, distribution, metabolism, and excretion of medications as well as other drugs. (This also applies to herbs.) The bottom line is that we need to understand the trade-off between the benefits of a medication and the costs of effects and side effects.

Poor Vision

Surprisingly, our eyesight can have a tremendous effect on our memory. If we do not see something in the first place, we will not remember it later. Therefore, we need to do our best to maximize our vision by getting regular eye exams and keeping our eyeglasses' prescription current. We also need to do all we can to reduce the likelihood of developing glaucoma and macular degeneration and of course wear eye protection when necessary.

Poor Hearing

Just as you can't recall something you can't see, if you don't hear what someone tells you, you cannot recall it later. I am 58 years old, but I have not yet had a hearing evaluation. Why not? How will I know if my hearing is making it harder for me to participate in the world and to hear and recall what I want and need to? Psychologically, it is so much easier to have an eye examination and to wear corrective lenses than it is to have an audiology evaluation and to wear hearing aids. I hope I don't wait until my wife is constantly telling me that the television is too loud to get a hearing evaluation and to use hearing aids, if I need them.

Alcohol

Alcohol causes forgetting. One domain of the memory research I have done was to evaluate the effects of alcohol on learning and memory in adults (young and healthy college students). Young adults who consumed alcohol clearly had poorer memory of newly learned information than did those who consumed a placebo. Interestingly, many were not able to reliably report whether they had consumed the beverage with alcohol or the placebo. The dose of alcohol used in the studies was below the legal limit of intoxication in most states.

If you enjoy your daily cocktail, beer, or wine, realize that it will impair your memory even if you do not feel the effects. Therefore, time your consumption of alcohol so it does not interfere with any important mental functions that require motor skills or memory. You also need to take into consideration that aging may cause alcohol to have a greater effect on mental and motor processes just as do many other drugs and medications.

Malnutrition

Malnutrition is another factor that makes mental operations less efficient and increases forgetting. Fortunately, I have not encountered this often in my work. However, there are cases where someone is very depressed or confused to the point that he or she cannot manage proper nutrition. This needs to be addressed since better nutrition will often cause afflicted individuals to think better. The effects of diet on memory in persons with normal nutrition are not well understood at this time. This topic will be addressed in chapter 12.

Fatigue

Fatigue contributes to forgetting. I am a morning (but not too early morning) person. This means that I will usually do better with all of my mental operations in the morning than in the evening. Others may be evening persons. They are more efficient at the end of the day. Know your patterns and plan more demanding mental activity during your peak times. If you get revitalized by taking a nap, do so. Take a walk to break up your work day and to make your mind more efficient and less fatigued.

Too Few Cues

As discussed above, clutter can inhibit memory and increase forgetting by adding interference (the enemy of primary and working memory). The inverse is also true. Having too few cues to trigger memory makes for increased instances of forgetting (transience and absentmindedness) that could have been avoided. Just leaving the umbrella beside the door would have saved me the cost of many umbrellas since I moved to Florida. It is extremely useful to have an environment rich in reminders of important things to do or to recall. A great deal of forgetting can be reduced by using external memory aids such as calendars, timers, other people, and tying recall to routine events (taking my morning medications when I shave). These aids will be discussed in Chapter 9.

CHAPTER SIX

Common Examples
of Memory Failure

Now that we have reviewed the concept of memory, the general effects of aging on mental processes, and common factors that increase forgetting, it is time to focus on what kinds of things are usually trouble spots for remembering. For example, when I give a seminar I provide a great deal of information. The problem is that most of us are not like S., and we cannot recall all of the details even an hour after the lecture, let alone ten years later.

One solution to this problem is to have this book. The information in the book is permanent, unlike spoken words. If you want to review a point, you merely need to go to the book and find the topic that you want to recall. Furthermore, if you attend the seminar and also read the book, you have spent more time and more effort with the material and are therefore likely to recall it better. You could also take notes of important points that you want to recall from either the seminar or the book to even further spend time with the information that you feel is important and further strengthen your memory for the material. In short, by knowing that the recall of details from lectures or speeches is transient, you can plan ahead to take steps to improve your memory by doing things like taking notes of points that you feel are important or tape recording the lecture for later review.

This chapter reviews several common examples of memory challenges for all of us. Anticipating these situations allows you to plan strategies and arrange the time necessary to improve your recollection and increase the strength of the memory you are forming. This is true for young adults with "normal" memory as well as adults who are experiencing the changes of aging. Knowing situations that are likely to challenge memory is even more important for those who have mild memory disorders and for those who care for them.

The major difference between those with mild to moderate memory disorders and those with "normal" memory is a matter of degree rather than of kind. So if we can anticipate where we may have memory challenges, we can set up systems to compensate for changes in efficiency to better prepare for those changes. This is like buying insurance. You buy insurance protection on your car before you have an accident and hope you will never have to use your policy. The same is true for managing memory. Good memory hygiene requires planning ahead. With this in mind, let's review some common areas that confront memory. It is also important to consider having a consultation and evaluation by a memory expert if you have any concerns about how your memory is working. This can allow you to more efficiently set up plans based on your own strengths and weaknesses.

Forgetting What Someone Tells Us

We often forget what someone tells us—this is especially true of details. If we could recall all of what is told to us, we would never have to take notes at lectures when we were in school.

Good note taking is a skill that requires planning ahead. It improves our memory both through the act of spending more time and effort with the information as we think and write and by providing an opportunity for future review of the notes.

VERBAL COMMUNICATIONS

We often forget what our spouses, friends, bosses, or colleagues tell us, at times much to our and their dismay. Of course, both the person telling you something and you must decide in advance what is important to remember. This way you will be able to spend more time and effort attending to and concentrating on the important parts of the message. This also allows you to make a few notes or mentally rehearse what is felt to be important.

As another example, in my line of work, I must recall many main details of what people tell me. I use notes to boost my recall, and my clients not only don't mind my making notes but often feel that I am taking them more seriously and listening better. As the consultations that I have are two-way communications, I suggest to my clients that they bring a tape recorder to sessions with me. Several of my clients have taken me up on this, and I make sure the machine is recording and place it on my lap or on a table close by. They can then later go to the tape to distill out what is important for them to recall and make notes before erasing the tape. This allows the client to spend more time and effort with the information that is helpful and to improve recall of important points.

Another good strategy for remembering what a person tells you is to be in the same room during the conversation and to talk face-to-face. I try to be especially careful to be in the same room with my wife or close friends when discussing important things and to repeat back to them what I think they told me in my own words. This allows me to clarify the communication, and it also allows me to spend more time elaborating my memory, which makes me less likely to forget what is important for me to remember.

DIRECTIONS

Remembering route directions that someone gives you can be quite challenging. This is true of even relatively simple directions. Listening to, recalling, and following directions places a large burden on short-term memory and attention. Getting and using driving directions is a complicated mental task that requires listening, driving, and navigating. There are so many things that can interfere with holding onto the directions, and it's even more difficult if you are tired or stressed. Personally, I am good for about two turns before I lose track if I try to hold directions in my memory. You can reduce a great deal of frustration and lost time by writing directions down or carrying a tape player.

PHONE MESSAGES

Phone messages are subject to quick forgetting as they also put a load on short-term memory. Don't rely on your ability to recall a message for a friend, a spouse, a colleague, or yourself. Write it down. Use this skill at home as well as at work. Have a pencil and paper next to the phone for writing down messages as they are being given. It may also be helpful to repeat the message back as this will reinforce your memory and make sure you have heard it correctly. Answering machines are also very helpful and can be used to replay the message as often as you need to.

REPEATED STORIES OR QUESTIONS

The longer I know someone, the more often I find myself telling them the same story. As I get older, I occasionally have more trouble keeping my place in conversation or knowing to whom I have said what. I also have more trouble recalling whether I said something or just thought it (misattribution or failure of source memory). I most often have these lapses when with my wife, friends, or colleagues with whom I spend a lot of time. It is also interesting how remembering and telling stories can transform the content of the story (encouraging suggestibility and bias). Each time information is recalled, my memory may be reconstructed by adding or subtracting information intentionally or unintentionally, thus changing what I say over time and repetition. I have not found a good strategy for helping manage this tendency. Others need to be patient with repetition. Telling stories serves a vital function to our well-being as will be discussed in the next chapter. Telling stories provides continuity in our life and allows us to enjoy the liberal use of long-term memory despite its tendency toward bias and distortion. This is especially true of anyone with a memory disorder.

One of the most stressful and aggravating aspects of living with someone with short-term memory loss (anterograde amnesia) is the repeated questions. Those with short-term memory loss cannot monitor what they have asked or not asked. Each time they ask a question, it is the first time for them. One way to reduce this is to keep track of repeated questions. This allows you to gain awareness of what is most often repeated. For example, I often encounter caregivers who are frustrated at being asked the date or what has to be done at a certain time (go to a movie) countless times during the day. This is a surefire source of loss of patience. In this case, a simple strategy can help. Simply have the person with memory loss wear a watch that has the date always available, and be sure he or she remembers to look at it. A good, easy-to-read calendar also helps to monitor what has to be done when and can dramatically reduce this repetition that results from a failure of prospective memory for time.

Difficulty Following Characters or Plot in a Novel or Movie.

I recently had a lunch conversation with friends who were older than fifty and had good memory. One of the participants mentioned that they were having more difficulty now than they used to following characters in a novel. This is especially true of novels with many characters and complex plots. This can also happen with movies or with TV shows that introduce new characters. Learning characters and plots (that is, new information) requires adequate short-term and working memory operations, which become less efficient with age and with disorders of memory.

If you enjoy reading, managing these changes is much easier than if you enjoy movies or television because you can go back to what you have forgotten. You can also list new characters or important facts as they appear in the text inside the front cover of the book, in a journal of what you are reading, and/or in the margins of the book. Underlining can also help because it allows you to spend more time with the item that you are rereading and helps you find the critical person or fact later. It's a good idea to include brief cues and page references for ease in looking up characters or facts later. Indeed, I have read many textbooks from my life as a student and a professional that are marked in the margins and front cover because I learned this strategy to help my memory when I started college. This facilitates learning the information in the first place because the process is more active than just reading. Furthermore, it allows me to focus on what I feel are the important facts or concepts during review, which further strengthens my memory. I continue to use this strategy today.

Another strategy that works well is to reread books, novels, or articles that you already have read. This allows you to use long-term memory rather than relying on short-term memory.

This becomes especially important for those who have difficulty with short-term memory. I worked with a client who loved reading science fiction but was having some mild short-term memory loss. She was very frustrated because she was struggling when reading new science fiction novels and was finding her favorite pastime frustrating rather than enjoyable and relaxing. She tried listing the characters but this no longer worked for her. As we discussed her frustrations, we decided to build on her strengths of long-term memory. She listed the science fiction works that she had on her bookshelves and wanted to reread sometime in the unplanned future. She proceeded to reread and greatly enjoy her favorite science fiction. This reduced her frustration and gave her more control. She is now marking the books she rereads that she most enjoys so she can read them again if her memory gets worse. The books she rereads will have the strongest memory traces and therefore be easier to follow because she is strengthening her long-term memory in an area that will bring her joy for years to come.

This strategy is more difficult for movies or TV programs that are current because they keep moving. Of course, you could tape the information that you wish to learn and later stop and review parts of the tape as needed. You could buy a DVD or videotape of the movie, when it is available, to review and be able to stop and take notes as desired or needed. Alternatively, you could focus your attention on movies or TV shows that you have enjoyed in the past as you are again exploiting your strength, your long-term memory. This may be the appeal of game shows on television. Game shows rely on long-term rather than short-term memory and can be enjoyed even by those with significant memory loss. This helps to explain the popularity of shows like *Jeopardy* or group games such as hang-man. Many who have short-term memory loss (even those with early and moderate Alzheimer's disease) can spend many enjoyable hours doing crossword puzzles, playing Scrabble, playing bridge, or watching old television shows that are now available on tape or DVD. This allows them to exploit their long-term memory and their personal history of interests and/or skills that can remain intact long into serious short-term memory loss.

Forgetting Names

The most common memory loss complaint is forgetting people's names. I have never had a good memory for names. I know that as I get older, this memory skill will not improve and will in fact probably decline. It often takes me three or four interactions with someone before I can master his or her name. I do much better recalling faces or specific information about the person than his or her name. Struggling to learn new names is another example of the aggravation that accrues with decline in short-term memory as a result of aging. It also represents the decline in our ability to bring to mind nouns, which is also a common memory problem as we age.

During lectures on memory, one of the first questions that people ask is how they can better recall names. This is true even for those who had a good memory for names earlier in their life. Names are especially problematic because they have so few associations; they are not "connotative" as pointed out by John Stuart Mill over a century ago. Names tell us little about the characteristics of the person. Consider what is called the Baker paradox. Think of someone named Mr. Baker. Now think of a person who works as a baker. Although we can try thinking about someone who works as a baker to remember Mr. Baker's name, there are probably very few actual associations of the person, Mr. Baker, to being a baker, especially if Mr. Baker does something for a living that is completely unrelated to being a baker. In other words, there are few or no connotative connections between the name and the person represented by the name.

Finally, many but not all of us have a skill that we could call being good at forming visual images. Those who have this skill have another strategy for learning and recalling names. For example, my name is "Bill." For some, this name could be more easily recalled by picturing the bill they will receive for consulting with me or imagining a duck's bill (the risk here is that they may call me Dr. Quack!). Of course, names such as Cotton, Greenfield, and Redman are easier to conger up images for than are names like Beckwith, Swenson, or Myers. This strategy of conjuring mental images to associate with names works much better where images are easy to come by.

Interestingly, we forgive others for forgetting our names but seem not to be as good at forgiving ourselves for not recalling the names of others. One strategy for managing memory for names is to be as forgiving of yourself as you are of others. I have often thought it would be helpful if we all had our name tattooed above our eyes. That way I could instantly make eye contact and know the name of the person with whom I am talking. More practical, though, is to use name tags whenever possible or construct a notebook with pictures and brief personal information on all those persons who are important to you. This allows you to study and review using not only language skills but also images, which takes advantage of multiple retrieval cues when you next encounter these people in the future.

Forgetting Where Things Are Placed

Another frustration that we all face is forgetting where things are placed (absentmindedness). (This, of course, does not apply to glasses. I am sure they have little hands and feet and crawl away when I am not looking.) We spend tremendous amounts of time hunting and gathering all those items we know we put *somewhere* that we could be spending in more enjoyable or productive pursuits. Forgetting where I laid down my keys has cost me more time than I would like to admit during my lifetime. It is also not a good idea to put things in a "special" but unique place so you will recall where they are; these items are often the ones we are most likely to be unable to find when we want or need them.

In principle, the solution for management of this failure of short-term memory is easy. Everything must have a place, and everything must be put in its place. The difficult part is that this includes the times when you are tired or busy or preoccupied, or just don't feel like it. This is an often-neglected skill that can save hours of time and frustration. It means placing your glasses in the same place every time, even when you are tired or it is inconvenient because you must walk across the house. The rule also holds true for portable phones, remote controls, and/or hearing aids. In terms of organizing important papers, this means establishing and then sticking with a specific filing system. The time you spend developing these skills and organizing your things will save you hours of time later.

Difficulty Learning a New Language or Learning New Motor Skills

Aging slows not only the learning of semantics (concepts) but also the rate of learning a new language or a new motor skill. An example of this is the learning of a second language. When I was in elementary school, it was not common practice for a second language to be taught. I also did not have the advantage of living near someone or having a relative who spoke a language other than English. I took three years of Latin in high school (though I can't recall any Latin). One of the requirements for obtaining my bachelor's degree was to develop a reading knowledge of a foreign language. (I took one year of French and two years of German.) All I recall from six years of language study are some syntax and structures of these languages. I never mastered any of them. It would have been so much easier on me if I had learned a second language as a child.

As another example of this principle in a different area, I did not learn to ski until I was in my 30s. It was very difficult for me to turn to the right (I am left handed), and I had to spend a great deal of time and effort to master movements to my right. The children in ski school appeared to struggle much less to master skiing. On the other hand, basketball was easier to master with my right side as I learned this skill in grade school. As we age, we need to plan on spending more time and effort if we are trying to learn a new skill. It is useful to break down new skills into small steps, and it often helps to have coaching or lessons to help you master the activity. It also helps to be persistent with frequent but short training sessions. These suggestions have helped many clients in their 70s and 80s master the computer, which is another skill that is not intuitive if you do not learn it when you are young.

Getting Lost

Getting lost can be very scary. Cities in coastal Florida seem especially challenging. Many of the cities have rivers and canals that cause challenges to route finding. It is very easy to get disoriented in these cities, especially if they are new to you. I have spent an inordinate amount of time driving around and trying to regain my orientation in these cities. A good map used to plan routes and identify directions before departing would have saved me a great deal of time and stress.

Although it is common to get lost in new places, it is not common to get lost in familiar places. This kind of getting lost or disoriented can be a sign of failing short-term memory or may be related to a neurological event such as a transient ischemic attack (a small or transient stroke). Routes and spatial maps are clearly stored differently by the brain than are oral directions. I do not have to "think" of the directions for most common places I travel. I once had a client who could give very good, detailed, and accurate verbal directions to all locations within the community where she lived. She could give directions to the bank, the activity center, the beauty shop, and the restaurants. She could also discuss in detail the experiences of her life and even compose music. However, she was unable to find any of the places she knew so well. She would get lost on the way to the bank that she had used so often over the years. She even had difficulty getting off an elevator and leaving her room.

It is always useful to get a good map of the area that you want to navigate and to learn the major streets and landmarks. When you plan to travel, you can study the map before you depart. You may also wish to draw a map of the route that you will take and carry it with you for reference. This extra time and effort of drawing the exact routes you will take on a separate sheet of paper may even keep you from needing to refer to the map during your journey. This allows you to spend more time and effort as well as to better reinforce the spatial map of your destination. It's important to also study the map and make directions for the return because the landmarks and turns are reversed and may confuse you. It may also be helpful to travel by day so you can more easily see the landmarks. It may also help to take along a navigator. If you are driving, these efforts will keep you from having to find the route and will also allow you to pay better attention to traffic, thereby making you a safer driver.

Forgetting Appointments, Birthdays, Medications

Forgetting appointments, birthdays, anniversaries, and medications are frequent memory complaints. Interestingly, several people who report this as a frustration say they do not keep a calendar anymore or never used a calendar in the past. They are concerned that they will weaken their memory by using "crutches" and therefore feel that they are helping to "strengthen" their memory by not using a calendar. These same people may have used a calendar at work but not at home as they "used to recall" the appointments they had and when they needed to be places.   Despite the rationalization that we are forgetting because "our mind is full," we need to be practical about appointments and important events that we want to remember in the future (prospective memory). This means keeping a detailed calendar. Put things on your calendar that you enjoy, such as vacations or times when friends or relatives are visiting or concerts you want to attend, as well as things you "need" to do, such as going to your dental or physician appointments. Include appointments with yourself to spend more time on your favorite hobbies or pastimes such as reading or bowling. Putting things that you enjoy in your calendar makes it more likely that you will do them. This is like a personal contract with yourself.

Having a good calendar habit is another kind of insurance that you can lead a relatively normal life even with short-term memory loss. Add to your calendar important birthdays, anniversaries, travel, or special events you want to remember, such as your exercise schedule. This prevents forgetting important upcoming events or people. As long as you refer to your calendar often and use it as a personal contract for your time, you can not only improve your memory, but you can also improve your social life and fitness and better manage your stress.

Medications may present another strain on our memory. For example, I need to take medications for high blood pressure. Therefore, it is an important for me to remember to take this medication reliably. I have developed the routine of leaving the bottle with my blood pressure medication next to my razor.

This way I have direct contact with the bottle each day as I shave, so I am not likely to forget to take the medication. However, for a time, I had to take the medication twice a day. It's amazing how much harder it was to remember to take a medication twice a day and how often I forgot. I knew I had forgotten by counting my pills at the end of the month. I had to establish a new routine for the evening medication because, as I mentioned earlier in the book, I was not reliable with the second medication despite my "trying" to remember. As we age, many of us need to take several medications, which increases the chances of forgetting or retaking medications.

The simplest first step in remembering to take your medications is to use a good pill organizer. Put the pill organizer in a place where you will reliably encounter it at the time of day that you need to take the medication. For example, if you need to take the medication at lunch time, keep the medication in the place where you eat lunch and make it stand out in this environment (put it next to your water glass). If you need to take the medication at a certain time of the day that does not have a natural marker, use a timer. Put the timer next to the medication container and use an alarm that will not stop annoying you until you see the container. In other words, the timer keeps making a sound until you mechanically turn it off. To further ensure reliability, keep a checklist of the times you take your medications to monitor how well your system is working. This way you will be able to discover any needs to further refine you system to reduce failures.

Forgetting That You Forget

An irony of anterograde amnesia, short-term memory loss, is that it causes you to forget that you forget. This is both a blessing and a curse. It would be very demoralizing to know all instances of forgetting. Forgetting that they forget is helpful to those with disorders of memory because it reduces their frustration. However, it also makes it more difficult for them to develop strategies to manage memory loss. Furthermore, this phenomenon can create a great deal of stress for those who live with a person suffering from significant anterograde amnesia. A recent case example illustrates this challenge.

We would all agree, even those with memory disorders, that there is a level of forgetfulness that makes it unsafe for someone to continue to drive. We probably also feel that we will know when our skills have deteriorated to the point that it is no longer safe to drive. Unfortunately, this is often not the way the situation unfolds. A client with moderate short-term memory loss recently reached the point where her family became aware that she could no longer safely drive. They had a very compassionate and lengthy discussion of the changes with her and made a plan for her to stop driving and sell the car. She had forgotten the discussion by the next day. After two months and several reminder discussions (each ending in her agreeing to the plan), she continued to forget the discussions. When confronted with selling the car, she became angry. She felt the decision was "out of the blue" and that her family was trying to sell the car for their own profit, despite the fact that she and her husband would have all of the money from the sale. The situation was finally resolved but only after a great deal of anger and repeated discussions. She obviously continued for some time to forget that she had forgotten.

One would assume that having a poor short-term memory would make you more likely to be insecure about facts and details that you "recall." However, this is often not the case. As short-term memory loss increases and becomes more severe, forgetting that you forget protects you from knowing that you have a poor memory. Many seem more likely to argue with others about facts they clearly recall incorrectly. If they can't find an item they are looking for and have misplaced, they may assume that the item was stolen. Managing this aspect of memory loss needs to be attended to before a person actually needs external memory supports, so it is important to learn to use external memory aids *before* you need them. They will be discussed in more detail in chapter 9.

I hope that I will anticipate my future memory needs as I grow older and that I will use many of the techniques from this chapter to make my memory better and reduce some of the frustrations that I and those close to me will encounter. If I or someone who knows me well is concerned about my mental operations or short-term memory, I hope that I will seek consultation with a memory expert to obtain an objective assessment of my memory. The feedback from such an assessment will help me and those who live closely with me to develop a plan and set up aids to manage my memory better, to monitor my memory over time, and to make progressive adjustments in the plan, if needed.

If my destiny is to develop a dementia, I must not be afraid of early detection of memory loss. If I develop good memory hygiene early in the course of memory loss rather than waiting until I am already demented, I will have the memory resources to do what is required. The major tools I will need are building on my long-term memory strengths, incorporating general rules of memory management, and developing my skills in using external memory supports. These tools will be discussed in the next three chapters beginning with a discussion of long-term and autobiographical memory.

CHAPTER SEVEN

Autobiographical and Long-Term Memory: *Who Am I and What Are My Skills?*

T o this point, the focus of this book has been on building an understanding of the varied forms and dynamics of memory. We reviewed the normal changes in memory that result from aging (inevitable alterations in efficiency that we must all manage as we grow older) as well as factors that increase the rate of forgetting, such as poor attention and distraction. On a broader level, the concept of memory

suggests that we are what we experience, and the more time we spend with our experiences, the better we will remember them.

Our life of experiences, knowledge, skills, interests, and self are the essence of long-term memory. Short-term memory is the process that allows experiences and information to be recorded or consolidated, relying on the brain system that is necessary for new learning. If short-term memory declines, as it does in Mild Cognitive Impairment or Alzheimer's disease, then we have increasing difficulty building long-term memory (even across a time period of minutes to hours). On the other hand, if short-term memory declines to the point that we develop anterograde amnesia, long-term memory becomes our strength. We retain our skills, knowledge, history, and our self, which allows us to function well in the world through considerable decline in short-term memory. Therefore, memory management must include an understanding of who we are, what we enjoy, what our skills and interests are, and what brings us joy. In short, we move forward, whether we have excellent or poor short-term memory, by going backward through the process of life review.

In the early 1960s, Robert Butler, a well-known gerontologist, defined life review as a universal psychological process triggered by the increasing awareness of our mortality as we age. Life review is more than a closing of our life; it is a universal consequence of life changes and transitions at any point in life. Life review is activated by events ranging from graduating from school, falling in love, getting married, moving, getting a job, changing jobs, or retiring from our job. Any life transition encourages us to review our life and redefine our sense of self. All of us are prone to review who we are and where we have been, so this process is not dependent upon becoming "elderly." Indeed, there are no significant differences between older and younger adults in frequency of reminiscing. Centenarians do not reminisce more often than adults in their 60s or 80s. Life review is not a sign of failing memory or health although it may be prompted by failing memory or health. Rather, life review is an adaptive response to life changes—it begins early and continues throughout life.

Functions of Life Review

Life review allows us to develop and maintain our sense of identity. It encourages us to appreciate ourselves and to understand our uniqueness. It can also help provide guidance for living our life and can empower our sense of continuity and purpose. Life review is an important component of our journey through life and relationships. It is especially important for anyone who is at risk of or has memory loss.

The skills and experiences that we store in long-term memory remain with us even as short-term memory loss progresses and as new learning becomes more and more difficult. We often hear that in Alzheimer's disease one cannot remember the present (what I ate for breakfast) but memory-impaired individuals can often recall with great clarity the past (how I stuck Susie's pigtails in the inkwell in third grade in 1932). It is true that short-term memory loss is a cardinal feature of Alzheimer's disease. However, as the disease progresses, there is also progressive long-term memory loss. But even in middle and late stage dementia there are islands of skills that may remain in long-term memory. For example, there are numerous cases of "demented" persons who appear apathetic and disinterested in the world about them. However, if they hear music that they have enjoyed and know well, they may get up and dance or sing along and appear to gain a momentary connection with the outside world that surprises those about them. Old pictures or movies may do the same thing.

Retelling our stories through life review is not always an accurate process, but it doesn't need to be. We all change the specifics of our stories as we tell them over and over. We recall the gist of events and may or may not accurately recall the details. For example, I recall visiting St. Augustine, Florida, when I was a child. However, the details of the city became quite distorted in my memory. When I visited St. Augustine in my early 50s, I was amazed at how poorly I had visualized and remembered the city. What I recalled of St. Augustine was actually a melding of other places both real and imagined. This process of transformation of memory over time, which includes mixing the details of one story with another, occurs more frequently in persons with Alzheimer's disease. They are even more likely than someone with normal memory to forget the facts from the past but to fill in details that either sound plausible to them or mix the details of different stories together. Of course only someone who knows them well would know the inaccuracies of the story. In other contexts we would refer to this transformation as creativity. The only difference, it seems, is the act of intention.

Even if stories become altered over time, we take for granted that we will be able to recall basic information such as our birth date, our husband's or wife's name, the names of our children, and the names of our grandchildren. However, those afflicted with Alzheimer's disease will become more vulnerable to forgetting their past and may even forget people who are extremely important to them. Having available resources like oral histories, video histories, photo albums, scrapbooks, and memorabilia can keep these memories alive for a much longer period of time for all of us, but especially for the person with memory loss. But these aids must be developed while long-term memory is still working fairly well. The process of developing these resources is enjoyable to anyone, whether they are young or old, whether they have good or poor memory.

The best time to review the past is now. We do not recall events better with the passage of time, even those of us with normal memory. Although it is critical that people who may have vulnerability to future memory loss (those with relatives who had a dementia, those who approach their 90s) organize and recreate their past, we can all benefit from the process of life review. Recreating the past is an important step in managing the distortions of transience, misattribution, and suggestibility. Recreating the past allows you to gain control of memory loss before it can occur and helps establish who you are and what is important to you. It defines skills that may be exploited if your memory declines.

It is important to create your life story in a concrete format. This can be done by simply organizing photos into albums or organizing memorabilia into scrapbooks. There are many books available that provide questions for you to answer about your life. You may hire a life historian to guide you through the process. If you are very ambitious and your memory works fairly well, you may wish to write your memoirs. The specific form is not important. Simple, brief, concrete formats are easier to create and to use.

Psychological Benefits of Life Review

There are also many psychological benefits of life stories. Creating a life history is an enjoyable process. Most of the clients I have worked with were skeptical when asked to meet with a life historian to complete a life history on audiotape. However, the intimidating tape recorder disappeared from consciousness quickly. The self-consciousness of talking about themselves also faded quickly, and participants often became lost in the process. Many have written notes thanking the historian for allowing them to have such an enjoyable time and stating how much better they appreciate who they are and the course of their life after spending about 90 minutes with a guide and a tape recorder. Most have listened to the tapes again and again, and many have given them to their children. Even the most reluctant (who usually stated that their life was too uninteresting to review) were pleased they completed this process.

Life stories and life reviews can be used clinically to alleviate depression, manage stress, and enhance self-esteem. Many of us are natural storytellers even though we may not be aware of it. We create our stories based on the stories of our parents, relatives, and models. We speculate about who they were and who we were at formative times in our lives. Life stories also can be used to stimulate thinking and enhance creativity, and to recreate interests or pleasures. We often get so involved in the routine of life, the errands, work, and keeping up the house, that we lose track of our interests.

Individuals with Alzheimer's disease have the additional burden of losing initiation. They do not spontaneously engage in activity or socialization. They often appear withdrawn and depressed. When asked what they used to enjoy, they may not be able to say because of the memory deficits. But if they have completed a life history that includes their interests, their life can be built around their uniqueness (called "biography-based programming"). This can be as simple as knowing that I love cats. Providing me with a cat can bring me endless hours of enjoyment. My cat will listen "attentively" to all of my repeated stories. My cat will never criticize or become frustrated with me. Knowing what music I like or dislike can also help provide me with joy in the present even if I develop a memory disorder.

Storytelling may even enhance the lives of those who already have moderate to severe memory loss. For example, my colleague formed a unique support group for couples who are struggling with managing dementia. One member of each couple has a dementia (ranging from very mild to moderate) and his or her spouse is the primary caregiver. This group has currently stayed together for two years with various structured activities including going on lunch outings, taking trips to museums, viewing videos, and playing games. As the group has continued, it is clear that the members with dementias show progression of their memory loss. The members of the group (those with normal as well as those with impaired memory) were asked at one point to be videotaped individually while telling some aspect of their life that they chose in advance of the taping. Even those with seemingly little participation during general group discussions were able to present a meaningful five-minute review of an aspect of their life that they chose. Everyone had a wonderful time when the tape was replayed, and this stimulated further reflection and discussion in all group members.

About a year later, several in the group were often silent and rarely participated in usual discussions. When they did speak, it was repetitious. Then all were asked to bring in a photograph of a grandparent. This was a "key" that opened up even silent members. All of the participants showed expressions of joy as they described their grandparent and the time they spent together. There is often much more inside persons with memory loss than we know. We need to find the keys to unlock what is there, and the keys are grounded in their histories.

Format and Structures for Life Review

There are many forms that life review can take. You can create an oral, pictorial, videotaped or written document, or a combination of two or more of these. You can engage in storytelling to a trained biographer or use a myriad of books that have questions to respond to. This process can be undertaken alone or with others in a group. No matter what the form, there are a few essential elements on which to focus in developing a personal history: birth, growing up, parents, siblings, school, work, marriage, children, grandchildren. One can also include places one has lived as well as travel, hobbies, interests, favorite books, lullabies, music, poetry, art, and pictures. All of these materials provide a rich and varied means (the keys) of providing comfort for anyone who completes the process, especially those with memory loss.

The more multidimensional and varied the format (use of words, images, photographs, creations) used in the re-creation of one's personal life story, the more beneficial it will be. The more coordinated the appearance, the more available the information is for review. We can establish who we are, what we enjoy, and in what areas we are skillful. This will then be available to us and others should our long-term memory begin to fail in the future. Planning ahead this way allows us to establish continuity in our life and relationships. Since long-term memory is reconstructive and fluid, your story should be told now. By creating your story now, you will provide yourself and others with potential clinical memory aids. If you wait until you *need* this information, you will not be able to develop it. Additionally, re-creating your life story provides intellectual stimulation and entertainment, and it makes concrete the legacy that you pass on to your family.

Although there are many possible structures for beginning to organize your life story, the following presents an outline of how to get started and some things on which you may wish to focus. The specific form you use is a matter of personal choice, taste, and convenience. Choose a format that is easy for you. Someone who is a skilled listener and knows when and where to ask questions can serve as a guide and help get you started. I have a professional life historian sit with my clients (those with good as well as those with poor memory) and spend about 90 minutes. During this time, she asks questions about their past starting with their places of birth, parents, and grandparents. The particular facets of history that gain focus depend on the person telling the story. The entire session is tape recorded (either with audio or video tape), and the tape is given to the storyteller at the end of the session. This is a very easy and enjoyable way to start the process. The product is a source of joy for the storyteller as well as for other family members.

There are many topics that you may wish to review. It is critical for those who may develop memory loss to include skills, talents and interests as well as family and important defining events in their lives. The following questions may serve as a guide to help with this process. Be sure to include reflections on important transitions such as childhood, adolescence, young adulthood, middle adulthood, school, college, military, marriage or primary relationships, role models, career, parenting, pets, or spirituality/religion.

1. FAMILY STORIES:
   What are the names of your grandparents?
   What was the country of origin of your grandparents?
   What are the names of your parents?
   What did your parents do for a living?
   What are the names of your siblings?
   What are the ages of your siblings?
   What was the birth order of the children in your family?
   Who are the important relatives that served as role models as you grew up?
   What are some of the earliest stories that you remember being told?
   What are your favorite family stories?
   What photographs or memorabilia best capture your family life?

2. SCHOOL STORIES:
   Who were your important teachers and mentors?
   What were your favorite subjects?
   Which subjects did you excel at?
   What are the shaping experiences from your elementary school?
   What are the shaping experiences from your high school?
   Did you attend college?
   Why did you choose that college?
   What was your major?
   Did you attend graduate school?
   Why did you choose that school?

What was your major?

What was your highest degree?

3. MARRIAGE STORIES:

How did you meet your spouse?

What attracted you to him or her?

How long did you date before you became engaged?

What is the date of your wedding?

Where did you get married?

How many years have you been married?

4. PARENTING STORIES:

If you have children, how soon after your marriage did you have your first child?

How many children do you have?

What is the name and date of birth of each of your children?

Where do your children live?

What kind of work do your children do?

How often do you see your children?

If you decided not to have children, how has this affected your life?

If you decided not to have children, how has this affected your relationship?

5. CAREER STORIES:

What was your first full-time job?

How did you get into your major life's work?

What have been the ups and downs of your career?

Is there another career that you wish you would have pursued?

How has retirement changed your life?

6. PET STORIES:
   Do you have a pet?
   What is your pet's name?
   What kind of pet do you have?
   What was your first pet?
   How does having a pet affect your life?

7. STORIES OF SPECIAL TIMES OR EVENTS:
   What is the role of music in your life?
   What is the role of art in your life?
   What is the role of literature in your life?
   What is the role of leisure and recreation in your life?
   What is the role of holidays and vacations in your life?
   What is the role of spirituality and religion in your life?
   What skills or things do you wish you would have
      learned?
   What do you do for exercise and how often do you
      do it?

CHAPTER EIGHT

General Rules
for Managing Memory

*Anything given less than
one minute of thought
will fade from your memory.*

– Douglas Herrmann,
author of *Super Memory* (1990)

B efore turning to specific techniques that help reduce the
memory flaws of transience, absentmindedness, and blocking, let's consider some general rules that assist us in understanding and managing our memory. These rules are not shortcuts to
a better memory. However, by attending to these principles,
you can better manage your efforts to increase the timing and
efficiency of your mental activity to better take in and recall
information. The next chapter provides the specific techniques
that focus your efforts on remembering.

RULE ONE: Memory Loss Cannot Be Cured

An issue keeps coming up in the professional as well as the pop-
ular press about memory. The issue is whether or not "mental
aerobics" or mental stimulation improves memory and/or prevents memory decline. As reviewed earlier, memory is a complex

and varied set of skills. Therefore, one cannot logically ask the general question of whether mental exercises improve "memory." Instead, the question needs to be asked relative to the *kind* of memory one wishes to improve. The answer to this question is different for the various kinds of memory reviewed in chapter 3: sensory, primary/working, short-term, and long-term memory.

Does practice or mental exercise strengthen sensory memory? As you may recall, sensory memory is the system that persists for only a part of a second (for example, the amount of time that you can hold the word you are currently reading before the next word displaces it). There are no exercises or types of stimulation of which I am aware that can strengthen sensory memory.

Does practice or mental exercise strengthen primary memory? Primary memory is the memory we use to remember a phone number before dialing it. It has an upper limit of information that can be held at any one time, which is about seven pieces of information. Primary memory remains active as long as we continue to rehearse or repeat these seven pieces of information. But primary memory is subject to interference by other information, such as an intrusive thought or the phone ringing. Practice and exercise cannot add capacity to this memory; it has only seven slots for most of us. But we may find ways to consolidate information to increase the data in each of those seven spaces. For example, we can "chunk" information. If we are trying to use this system to hold a phone number, we can take advantage of common prefixes, such as remembering that all numbers at work start with the prefix 454. This uses only one of the slots rather than seven, so we have two extra slots with this technique. We can also make use of patterns to help make primary memory more efficient. For example, the numbers 1234 or 2468 are easier to recall than is the number 9253 because the former can be more easily grouped by a pattern, thereby opening up more of the slots available. In short, cleverness can make more efficient use of the seven spaces, but exercise does not make primary memory stronger.

Does practice or mental exercise strengthen short-term memory? This is the memory system that keeps information for minutes to hours. It is the system that manages, sorts, and manipulates information. Short-term memory is also the process or system that permits consolidation or storage of information into long-term memory. This is the memory system that is impaired in disorders of memory such as Mild Cognitive Impairment and Alzheimer's disease. As discussed in previous chapters, weakness in short-term memory produces anterograde amnesia, making it difficult to learn new information. Unfortunately, this memory system does not function like a muscle, which increases in strength with repetition or practice. Therefore, mental stimulation and mental exercises do not make short-term memory stronger. Many suggest that exercises such as learning to write with your nondominant hand or learning to do crossword puzzles will improve your memory or prevent or delay the onset of Alzheimer's disease. However, short-term memory does not respond to exercising it any more than we can strengthen our eyesight by not wearing our glasses.

But mental exercises and stimulation *do* strengthen long-term memory. The "use it or lose it" principle clearly applies to long-term and procedural memory but does not work for short-term memory. While short-term memory can't be improved, the good news is that it can be managed through the use of specific techniques that will be discussed in the next chapter.

RULE TWO: Make Use of Your Remaining Skills and External Memory Aids

If you feel that your memory—that is, your short-term memory—is not as good as it used to be, make use of other skills such as good organization. It's a good idea to build your arsenal of memory supports early. If you cannot keep track of the date and the day of the week reliably, use a digital watch to compensate. If you forget what you are to do during the day, take a daily "to-do list" with you so you know what to do and when to do it. It may also help to seek consultation with a memory expert to help determine particular strengths and weaknesses of your memory. This will allow you to make use of the best strategies for you.

It's important to understand that external memory aids are not crutches. Rather, they allow you to more efficiently use your remaining skills, much like wearing eyeglasses. Many have said to me that they should not use external memory aids, such as calendars or digital watches, because these "crutches" will further weaken their memory. This is simply untrue. I have used a calendar to track my time for years. This does not mean that I am weakening my memory; it means that I am trying to be clever in managing my memory and not forgetting many things that are important to me. Building a good calendar habit clearly benefits my memory, but it does take me more time and effort than merely "trying" to remember.

RULE THREE: **Keep Learning Sessions Short and Frequent**

The best way to learn new information (things we want to or must remember) is to learn it in small bits and repeat it often. This is the same principle we all learned in school. Cramming for an exam is both inefficient and unreliable. Frequent, short, spaced study sessions build much stronger long-term memory. It is much easier to learn two new names than it is to learn ten. You can master the other eight (preferably a couple at a time) after the most important two are recalled reliably.

RULE FOUR: **Manage Stress**

We all experience stress. So far, no one has found a way to eliminate stress, and I am not sure that this would be as good for us as it sounds. Indeed, it may be that having no stress would reduce motivation and impair learning, resulting in little need for memory. We may operate best under moderate levels of stress, which add to motivation and effort. It is the high (panic) and low (nearly asleep) levels of stress that are disruptive to learning and memory. Techniques to help manage stress will be discussed in chapter 14.

RULE FIVE: **Reduce Distraction**

Make your environment work for you rather than against you. Turn off the television. Do the most demanding mental work when you are rested and efficient, which is the mornings for many but not all of us. Turn off the phone and let the answering machine take messages while you are working. If you want to recall what someone is telling you, be in the same room, make eye contact, and repeat the message back in your own words.

RULE SIX: **Spend More Time and Effort**

The more time you spend with something, the better you learn and recall it. Old skills get "rusty." This is where "use it or lose it" works. We remember best the information with which we spend the most time. New information does not stick if you do not spend enough time with it and make an effort to learn.

RULE SEVEN: **Repeat and Practice**

Long-term memory, knowledge, and skills are built on repetition. This is a part of the effort that we must expend if we are to better manage our memory. You may not learn someone's name unless you repeat the name upon first meeting the person or see the same person in multiple situations.

Practice is building a routine to systematically repeat things you want to learn or to keep current information or skills that you don't want to fade. The more often you do something, the better you become at it as a result of better memory. Therefore, it's a good idea to schedule regular practice sessions to keep skills and information that you want to retain available and efficient. Great musicians and artists become great only by constant repetition and systematic practice. Their skills and memory fall off if they do not put time into their craft.

RULE EIGHT: **Make Associations**

Memorizing by rote is very difficult. For example, if I ask you to remember three-letter sequences that are not real words, such as cqz or kyc, you will find that they are very difficult to learn and recall. On the other hand, if I ask you to recall a sentence such as "The hiker climbed the tree," you can use images or associations to assist with learning and later recalling. For instance, to recall this sentence, you might visualize a bear at the base of the tree that chased the hiker, who climbed up the tree for safety. It becomes much easier to recall the sentence at a later time both because you spent more time and more effort in learning the sentence in the first place and because you now have an association or cue to trigger the memory later. This example lends itself well to forming a visual image that further increases the likelihood that you will recall the sentence at a later time.

RULE NINE: **Organize**

People who are well organized are much more likely to remember what needs to be done when. They also save much time and effort that those of us who are not as well organized expend on looking for things and simply handling materials over and over that we plan to deal with at some unidentified future time.

I must admit that I am a "stacker." I have many piles of "stuff" that I feel I need to attend to eventually. I often let my piles accumulate over long periods of time, and each pile is somewhat eclectic. I don't allocate enough time to organize the things I have to do into files that I could more easily use. I do not keep a "to do" list where I can realistically decide what can be done in a day and cross off items as they are completed, which would be a good reinforcer for me. I do not use my calendar to schedule time to make necessary phone calls. In short, I am not a good organizer. I would "forget" fewer things and have to make many fewer apologies for not being timely if I would spend more time and effort to get organized and to stay organized.

RULE TEN: Engage in Relaxation at Least One Time Each Day

Spending at least some time each day in formal relaxation has been shown to enhance performance on professional memory tests as we age. This suggests that relaxation may enhance memory in everyday situations as well. Relaxation is one way to manage stress. It allows the emotions to "cool off" at least once a day. A friend told me that one of the most productive things he did each day at work was to take a short nap. Another friend turns off the phone, props up his legs, turns down the lights, and meditates each day after lunch. These are routines that we could all benefit from for improving our mental efficiency and memory as well as reducing our stress. There are a multitude of ways to engage in relaxation. You can obtain tapes or work with a therapist who can train you in relaxation skills. You can learn meditation or yoga, both of which are great ways to induce a relaxed state. The important thing is that you (and I) need to organize our lives in such a way that we can provide ourselves with a period of relaxation at least once a day.

CHAPTER NINE

Techniques That Work to Manage Memory

W*hat can I do to improve my memory?* By now I'm sure you realize that this is not the right question. If you want to improve your short-term memory, you need to manage new information (associate with the familiar and common, use cues, arrange your environment), manage forgetting, and manage attention. If you want to improve your long-term memory, start by managing your short-term

memory, then practice, rehearse, and review regularly. Long-term memory accrues and is strengthened by exercise; short-term memory is not affected by exercise.

Recall the extreme examples provided by H.M. and S. H.M. demonstrated severe short-term memory loss, anterograde amnesia. His memory loss was much more severe than is found in most cases of Alzheimer's disease. He could not learn new people, places, or events. Yet his long-term memory, prior to 1951, remained very good. On the other hand, S. could remember it all. He demonstrated what is called extreme hypermnesia. S.'s short-term memory was too good. Fortunately, most of us do not have to live with either of these memory problems.

Short-term memory does not itself learn. Rather, short-term memory promotes learning through allowing consolidation to occur. Short-term memory in coordination with working memory allows sorting, selection, association, and rehearsal so that we can move information to long-term memory. Long-term memory is the reservoir of learning and is what most mean by the term memory. Long-term memory consists of facts, skills, knowledge, and self. The challenge we all face is how to better manage short-term memory. Long-term memory usually takes care of itself as long as we manage our short-term and working memory and we revisit and review what we feel is important.

Many memory courses over the years have relied on training in techniques called mnemonics. These techniques date back to a time before writing was convenient (before the invention of printing presses, let alone computers). Mnemonics were designed for orators who passed on oral traditions that required memorizing extensive narrative. An example of a mnemonic is the "peg" method (this is also known as paired associate learning). If you want to recall items to buy at the grocery store, for example, you associate them with a predetermined set of elements such as the clothing that you are wearing. To remember to buy bread, butter, eggs, and salmon, you might pair bread with your shirt, butter with your pants, eggs with your socks, and salmon with your shoes. This makes use of long-term and short-term memory. The problem with this and other classical mnemonic techniques is that few people use them spontaneously, and they are less and less likely to be used as we age. Even those trained in these methods don't often use them in everyday life. Finally, persons with short-term memory loss cannot learn the techniques, and those who already have learned them will probably quit being able to use such complex methods. Still, a few mnemonic techniques are simple enough to help us manage our short-term memory, so I have included these below.

What we all need are reliable, simple methods that help us better manage our mental resources and efforts. This in turn will improve our long-term memory. Such techniques can orchestrate short-term memory and boost long-term memory. These techniques reduce the load on primary and short-term memory and take advantage of skills we already have. The techniques described below will help you to remember better whether you are 20 or 90. You can choose from this list the techniques that best suit your own memory needs. However, some of these techniques, such as a good calendar habit, are essential to nearly all of us.

Name Badges

One of the most typical frustrations of many is recalling names. Names present a challenge for short-term memory. Names are usually first presented in a single introduction and have few natural associations. If you are distracted, as may often be the case when meeting someone new, interference will remove the name from primary memory even before it has a chance to get into short-term memory. That's the reason for the common suggestion of repeating the name during your greeting when you first meet someone new, saying, "It's nice to meet you, Bob," rather than merely saying, "It's nice to meet you." A simpler method is to wear a name badge. This gives a person meeting you the opportunity to rehearse your name easily and make multiple associations between your name and your face. Name badges are simple and very reliable ways to recall names.

Flash Cards

Flash cards are a technique that we often used in school but do not usually generalize to other times in our life. Any information that must be learned, such as vocabulary or names, can be organized onto flash cards for easy study and review. The act of making the cards also helps you spend more time and effort with the information to build stronger memory traces from the start. Many of the students with whom I have worked used flash cards to help prepare and study for exams. As another example, I provide each participant of small groups that I conduct with pictures and names of everyone in the group so they can more easily study and learn names of other group members.

Notebooks

Notebooks are fundamental examples of the benefits of organization. The mere act of making the notebook utilizes short-term memory to promote rehearsal and facilitates review, thus allowing for stronger long-term memory. The act of making the notebook automatically makes you spend more time and effort with the information and often utilizes multiple images (written words, pictures). Making a notebook for each course I took was one of the memory skills that helped me get through many years of education. I kept notes from lectures and readings in notebooks organized by subject. I usually rewrote class notes the same day as the lecture. This allowed me to review information while it was fresh in my mind to help promote better long-term memory of information over which I would later be tested. Computers and palm-sized organizers make notebooks even easier to construct today for those who are comfortable with computers. For important projects, I still take written notes and make notebooks to organize and review information.

A memory notebook is a specialized notebook that is structured to organize what we are concerned that we might forget into an easily usable format. Memory notebooks are especially useful for anyone who has short-term memory loss. The notebook could contain information such as the medications that you take and your medical history, which can be very useful for physician visits, especially with physicians whom you have not seen before. Or a memory notebook can be used to track what you want to remember to do, such as errands. Memory notebooks work best when they are well organized and brief, focus on currently important information, and are carried with you at all times. The information included will depend on what you feel you need and want to remember and what you are likely to forget.

Journals

A journal is a record of events, transactions, and observations that is kept at frequent intervals. This is a wonderful memory aid for keeping track of one's life. For example, you may want to keep a journal(s) of vacations and trips. If you are a movie buff, you may wish to keep a journal of movies that you have seen and basic facts about the movies that you want to recall, such as the names of the movies and actors in roles. How often have you forgotten details of a trip or movie that you enjoyed and would like to recall? Alternatively, you might keep a journal on the places that you have lived during your life. Reviewing journals allows you to revisit things that you have enjoyed. Journals also help sustain long-term memory by providing easy review, promoting reminiscence, and serving as documentation of your interests and pleasures.

Diaries

A diary is very similar to a journal but usually contains more personal reflections or feelings about events, situations, people, and times. Of course, diaries may be combined with journals of important information, events, transactions, and observations. Journals and diaries take time and effort to create, but they are an excellent means of organizing information that is felt to be important and are also a good source of review.

Calendars

Nearly everyone uses some kind of calendar to keep track of important things to do such as appointments. For most this means having a master calendar at home that contains many details over long periods of time (weeks or months). However, the most detailed and wonderful calendar that is at home when you are not does you no good. To make your memory more reliable, it is helpful to carry a daily calendar or appointment book with you. The most useful daily calendars are organized into days with times and enough space to write. In my case, I often wish I had my daily calendar "leashed" to my person so I would not misplace it or forget to bring it.

The effort taken to construct a daily calendar or appointment book anew for each day helps to build a stronger memory of what you want to accomplish during the day and may make it less likely that you will even need to refer to it (assuming that you have an adequate short-term memory). The daily calendar aids your attention as it reduces interference from what you did the day before or what you have to do tomorrow. Your master and daily calendars should contain pleasant events or things you want to do as well as things you "have" to do. For example, you can schedule time to listen to music, read, walk, and enjoy conversations and intimate time with your mate or close friends. Include the movies, concerts, or plays you want to see as well as important birthdays and anniversaries to remember. Include your exercise and stress management routines. You could even use your appointment book to remember to send flowers to someone you love "spontaneously" on a predetermined but regular schedule.

One of my clients and her husband use her calendar in a very creative way. She has mild short-term memory loss but a very good calendar habit that she developed before she experienced memory loss. Her calendar is the blueprint for her to keep her life together as her short-term memory declines. One of the frustrations that she developed with memory loss was doing laundry. The couple ran out of clothes before she would remember to do the laundry again. If she did start the laundry, she forgot to move the clothes from the washer to the dryer. And the clothes could remain in the dryer for a week because she would not remember to take them out. Her husband decided to help, but this led to conflict because she felt strongly that doing laundry was her job and doing it made her feel good about herself. After discussing her frustrations, we devised a plan where she would do laundry on Saturdays. She brought her master calendar and we entered "put laundry in the washer" at 9:00 a.m., "put the clothes in the dryer" at 9:30 a.m., and "remove the clothes from the dryer" at 10:30 a.m. This was added to her schedule on the calendar for every Saturday for the rest of the year. Both she and her husband felt this plan worked very well. They always had clean clothes, and they no longer had to argue because she felt bad about not being able to do the laundry without his assistance.

Address Books

Address books are another specialized journal and may include phone numbers and addresses that you want or need to remember. Keep your address book up-to-date and neat for easier use. It can be very difficult to decipher entries in an address book where there are many items crossed off or written over.

To-Do Lists

To-do lists force us to decide what is important to complete. They also help us to set goals and to reinforce our efforts by allowing us to see our progress. To-do lists should be revised often and work best when they are neat and organized. Having many crossed off items and scribbles interferes with attention and increases rather than decreases memory failures. Items should be crossed off as they are completed. It also helps to make a new list each day. The items placed on the to-do list should be realistic and manageable in a short time period, such as a day. It may also be helpful to have larger goals broken down into a series of brief sub-goals or steps. These lists keep you from forgetting what you want to accomplish as well as allowing you to better manage stress by concretely seeing your progress toward both short- and long-term goals.

Grocery Lists

Grocery lists are specialized to-do lists. Despite the fact that they can save a lot of time and aggravation, I don't often see people working from lists at the grocery store, and I often do not use a list. But I have also made many extra trips to the store because of items that I have forgotten to buy when I didn't use a list, and there are many other ways I would rather spend my time. A grocery list saves time and makes you less likely to forget. The list works especially well if you organize it by categories of foods and check off items as you put them in your cart.

Taking Notes

Taking notes is another skill that we all had to master to survive in school. Taking notes helps support short-term memory and is an aid to build long-term memory. Writing main ideas down allows you to review what you were told or what you read. The act of taking notes makes you spend more time with new information. Furthermore, taking notes encourages you to ask questions to clarify things about which you may be unsure. Although taking notes is an obvious way to recall phone messages and conversations, surprisingly few of the clients who come to me for advice about how to improve their memory have a note pad and pencil next to their phone. In addition to writing down phone messages, it is also helpful if you read back to the caller important information that you have noted to be sure it is correct. Reading back also adds repetition, which builds long-term memory.

Tape Recorders

Tape recorders provide us with an often neglected yet simple way of managing memory. For example, you may wish to take a tape recorder with you for your next visit to your physician. This way you will be able to recall what he or she tells you, and you can also review explanations, instructions, or changes that may be recommended. Critical information can later be transferred to a journal organized around medical information. Alternatively, you may wish to record lectures or talks by others that you feel are important. You can later select and transfer this information to a more easily accessible format such as a journal or notebook. There are many types of tape recorders that can be used for special purposes. For example, one of my clients bought a small recorder (about the size of a half dollar) that was on the ring that she attached to her keys. Whenever she parked her car, she recorded its location and saved herself hours of time and frustration that she had previously spent looking for her car after coming out of the malls or grocery stores. And her clever system had the recorder on the chain with the car keys as a cue to use it.

Timers

It is interesting that we are accustomed to using an alarm clock (a timer) to arise in the morning, yet many are resistant to using a timer to mark time for other events during the day. We try to remember to take medications at specific times, to monitor cooking while involved in other pursuits, to remember to take the clothes out of the dryer. Trying doesn't work well; timers do. Timers can even be used to help you remember to look at your calendar. Timers can be very helpful in developing new routines such as remembering to exercise at a certain time or to engage in relaxation each day. They can also be used to remind you when to leave to go to a movie or a play that you don't want to be late for. You can even use timers to prompt you to make phone calls. In short, timers are very good for prospective recall, that is, recalling that you need to do something at a preselected time or interval.

Clocks and Watches

We organize so much of our time by clocks that we take them for granted. Modern clocks can do much more than just tell time. For those who are comfortable with computers, the clock in the computer can be used as a timer to track medications, personal schedules, and things to do. Computers can also remind you to look at your calendar. For those who are not comfortable with computers, the alarms in watches or clocks can remind us to look at a calendar or take a medication at critical times. Many digital clocks can now be used to assist in keeping track of date, day of the week, month, and year. We never have to be disoriented in relation to time as long as we have a good clock or watch that contains this information. Some clocks are even updated for time and date every day as a satellite passes by and are therefore always accurate. I love my "atomic" clock in the bedroom. It is always accurate, and it is one less clock to remember to reset when the time changes in the spring and fall. Digital clocks work from batteries, so they aren't influenced by interruptions in power. They can even indicate when the batteries need to be replaced.

For those with short-term memory loss, using digital watches is imperative. They are unlikely to be misread and allow you to always be oriented to time. The display should be easy to read and have critical information displayed at all times without the need to switch functions. Watches and clocks can also be found that present time and date aloud. These watches and clocks were developed for those with failing vision but can be helpful to anyone who finds them convenient.

Pagers

A pager is a specialized timer that you or someone else can use to remind you to do things such as make a phone call, exercise, or take medications. One of the clients I worked with had a unique problem. He had severe pain from arthritis that caused him to have difficulty getting going in the mornings. He had to wait for the pain medication to start working before he could move after awakening. He had the additional problems of being severely hearing impaired without his hearing aids (he did not sleep with them) and having severe macular degeneration that limited his functional vision. As we discussed his frustrations, it occurred to us that a good solution was to have him awaken to take his pain medications a couple of hours before he wanted to awaken for the day. We used a pager set on vibrate that he wore at night against his skin. This woke him so he could take the medication, after which he returned to sleep. This system worked very well for him.

Pillboxes

We have increasingly become a pill-taking culture. It seems that a normal part of aging in contemporary America is taking medications. Many of these medications, such as cardiovascular and diabetic drugs, have significantly added to the general life span and quality of life. But the successful use of medications requires memory, especially if you have to take multiple medications. The main tool for reliable use of medications is a pillbox, and some of these have useful bells and whistles.

The most reliable and easy-to-use pillbox is a device that sits in your house and is connected to a computer over your phone line. Each time you need to take a medication, the pillbox sounds an alarm which does not stop until you open the compartment with the pill and take it out. If you fail to open the compartment within a certain time, you will receive a phone call reminding you to take the pill. This pillbox would be very good for someone with anterograde amnesia. While many pillboxes are much simpler and less expensive than this one, the most helpful pillboxes are those that make a sound when the pill needs to be taken and don't stop making the sound until the pillbox is opened.

In addition to a good pillbox, it is also important to match medication times with events that you always complete and to keep the pill organizer in the space where you complete those tasks. For example, if you wash your face at 8:00 each morning, keep your pillbox on your sink. If you brush your teeth each evening before going to bed, keep your evening pillbox by your toothbrush. To be sure that you are reliable in taking medications, it is also helpful to have a monitoring system such as a checklist to assess your accuracy.

Walkie-Talkies

Walkie-talkies can serve as a pager as well as allowing two-way communications. Although they are commonly used in some workplaces, they can also be useful in places like airports and shopping malls to keep contact with someone. Walkie-talkies can be a convenience for anyone, but they are especially useful for couples when one of the spouses had short-term memory loss. One of the most vulnerable situations for these couples is bathroom breaks either in a shopping mall or at an airport. I know of several instances in which the couple became separated, and the person with memory loss tried to find his or her spouse, only to become lost. This causes fear and anxiety for both people. An easy solution is to use walkie-talkies in these situations as they allow contact to be made and finding the other person fairly easy. Although cellular phones can also serve this function, cellular phones are more complicated to use, especially for anyone who may have mild memory loss and was not familiar with using cell phones before the decline.

Computers

Computers are major and complex external memory systems. They are becoming increasingly used to quickly track and store information. Computers contain schedules, timers, encyclopedias, diaries, calendars, etc. They can manage the simple as well as the complex. They may be large (desktop) or small (laptop). They can be portable, such as a laptop or a palm-sized organizer. They can be so small that they can be held in your hand or even worn on your wrist as a large watch. (Dick Tracy lives!) Many modern telephones, especially cellular phones, have computer functions, as do many televisions.

Computers are wonderful and reliable aids for managing memory. But to take advantage of computers requires that you be comfortable with their use. A daughter of one of my clients sent her mother a computer to assist her with failing short-term memory. However, her mother did not like the computer on her table and was always intimidated by the machine, which she called the "beast." Needless to say, this computer never helped the woman better manage her memory. Another factor to consider is that one of the signs of early mental decline can be loss of abilities such as being able to use the programs that your have already mastered on a computer. I have had several computer-literate clients who knew they were having memory troubles because they could no longer use all of the programs they knew on the computer. In several cases we were able to devise checklists that were placed near the computer in a notebook to help manage this frustration for them.

Organized Work Space

Clutter interferes with attention which, in turn, interferes with memory. It is therefore extremely helpful to reduce clutter and organize in order to better manage your memory. One important key to organizing a work space is to keep out only active projects. Other projects should be organized but kept out of the active work space. Another key to organization is to make your priorities and stick with them. Eliminate things that you have not "gotten to" in weeks. Chances are that if you have not gotten to something within six months, it has low priority. Keeping it around to worry about will simply interfere with other, more urgent projects and tasks.

The best use of this technique of organizing a work space that I have seen was that of a client who had suffered a traumatic brain injury. She loved to cook but found that after the injury she could no longer complete recipes without leaving out items. Her solution was to organize all items for the dish she was cooking on the counter in the order she would use them. She then worked from one end of the counter to the other. If there was any interruption, she cleared the counter, set up all items again, and completed the preparation of the food. She was very pleased with this routine and said it saved her a great deal of frustration and put the joy of cooking back into her life.

Routine Placement of Objects

Everything has a place, and everything must always go in its place. This may sound obvious and simple, but it can be very difficult to follow. It takes good organization and planning, and you must spend time initially setting up places for things. Routine placement of keys, glasses, hearing aids, and important papers saves even those with normal memories a great deal of time. Portable phones and TV remote controls are sources of a great deal of search-and-find time. Many televisions and phone have devices allowing you to push a button so the phone or remote will beep to help you find it. You can also find these devices for small objects, such as your keys, but you must always be able to easily find the main remote to send the signal to the receiving alarm, so the rule of routine placement of objects applies even to these devices.

The key to this memory technique is that everything must go in its place no matter how inconvenient, no matter how tired you may be. One of my clients used this method to take her sunglasses with her when she went outside. She was continually frustrated by forgetting her sunglasses, so we decided to have her place a small shelf at eye level next to her door. She made a habit of placing her sunglasses on the shelf as she entered her apartment, and she never forgot to take her sunglasses with her again.

Take-Away Spot

How can I remember to take everything I need each day when I leave the house to go to work? I have often gotten to work and left something behind. To compensate for this, I use a take-away spot by the door to the garage. I keep all items that need to go with me when I leave in the morning in a box in that spot. The take-away spot is a specific example of routine placement of objects.

It is very important to place items that will need to go with you in the box or spot as you think of them. Any delay because it feels like too much effort, it seems inconvenient to go to the box at the moment, or you are too tired increases the likelihood that you will leave without that item. I have even used this with umbrellas. I often will leave my umbrella on the door handle or next to the door if I am visiting someone. This has reduced the number of umbrellas that I must buy every year.

Travel Souvenirs

Travel souvenirs such as trinkets, postcards, photographs, slides, and refrigerator magnets are concrete objects that can supplement journals and diaries in keeping your memories of pleasing times. Refrigerator magnets are excellent ways to be reminded of your favorite places and favorite trips. Souvenirs help keep valued experiences easily available for later recall, reminiscence, and enjoyment.

Visual Imagery

Visual imagery is a more complicated strategy for memory management. Some of us are naturals at forming images whereas others are not. We all can better recall objects that can be formed into an image. We all know people who can picture in their head what a room will look like painted a certain color or with a new sofa. If you have this skill, exploit it by trying to form images of objects that you wish to remember. I was once testing the memory of a very clever artist by reading her a long list of words. She looked around the room and visualized objects in the room that were on the list. This greatly enhanced her score on the testing of those words that had representations in my office, for example, bookcase. Some things are easier to translate into an image than are others. It is easier to recall a table or a bookcase than it is to recall a concept such as anger or knowledge. Unfortunately, imagery requires skills and effort that are not often available to those with significant short-term memory loss.

Elaboration

Elaboration is another complicated strategy for enhancing memory by spending more time with important things that we want to learn or recall. For example, if you are trying to recall the names of several landmarks that allow you to travel a new route, you might list the landmarks and create a story that links them. Alternatively, you might attach the landmarks to items of clothing that you are wearing. These strategies allow you to have structure around which to learn and remember new information.

Rhymes and Jingles

Rhymes are a specialized example of elaboration. Rhymes have been used as a mnemonic technique for as long as oral information has had to be recalled. Rhymes are a mainstay of advertising. For example, what comes to mind when you see a check mark or hear the slogan "just do it?" If you are old enough, try to complete the following sentence, "See the USA in your _____." Again, this takes a great deal of effort and may not work very well for many with short-term memory loss.

PQRST

PQRST (preview, question, read, state, test/review) is another technique that we used in school but often don't apply to other parts of our life. This method takes a great deal of effort and time and is used by students to enhance studying and learning new information. It is usually applied to learning from textbooks but could be applied to any written material that you wish to better retain. This is an active rather than a passive method of reading that helps to build better long-term memory by incorporating repetition and review early in the process of learning.

PREVIEW
Before reading an article in a magazine, browse through the article. Note pictures, captions, subheadings, summaries, and abstracts. This starts to create a map in your mind of the information that will be learned and begins to build a memory trace.

QUESTION
For each heading, ask a question anticipating what you will read and want to learn from the material.

READ
Read the material of interest.

STATE
Answer your questions in your own words as you read the material.

TEST/REVIEW
Use the questions to later test your memory of what you have read and to help you know what facts or concepts you need to spend more time with.

Expanding Rehearsal

Expanding rehearsal is a simple yet effective way to learn small bits of new information. For example, if you wanted to learn a new word that was difficult for you to remember, you could use this technique. Let's say you wanted to learn the word "mnemonic" (a technique to assist with memory). Start by saying "mnemonic." Then wait 30 seconds and say "mnemonic" again from memory. Next wait 60 seconds to repeat the word. Double the retention interval each time you repeat the word until you can easily recall the new word. If you miss recalling the word at a certain interval, go back a few intervals and build the time between recalls without making a mistake again.

I had a client with short-term memory loss who kept forgetting the name of a grandchild who was getting married. It was important to him to go to the wedding and be able to recall his grandchild's name. He used this technique for two weeks before the wedding and was successful in his goal. Expanding rehearsal could also be useful for recalling new names or for learning vocabulary words in a foreign language. This technique requires a lot of effort, but it can be a very effective way to build a new memory.

Fading

Fading is another technique for new learning that requires a great deal of effort but is very effective. To learn about this technique, try using the following cues to help master the spelling and recall of the word "mnemonic." At each step, say the word out loud and spell it upon seeing the written-out visual cue. As you can see, each successive step presents less information (one less letter from the end of the word) to stimulate memory of the word and its spelling. You could further reinforce learning the word by using it in a sentence, which is the method of elaboration.

"Mnemonic"

"Mnemoni"

"Mnemon"

"Mnemo"

"Mnem"

"Mne"

"Mn"

"M"

Search Mnemonics

Search mnemonics are simple strategies that often help cue memory when spontaneous recall fails. These techniques are especially useful for nouns/names.

FIRST LETTER OR NUMBER

Try to think of the first letter of the name or noun that you want to recall, or the first number of a longer number you need to recall. This often primes association networks and allows you to recall names and numbers. For example, if I momentarily cannot think of my phone number, I might think that it starts with a 4, which might cue the prefix 454 and then the rest of the number.

ALPHABET SEARCH

This is a similar strategy. Start reciting the alphabet to try to come up with the first letter of a name you are trying to recall. My name comes quickly if this works—Bill. If my name were Zena, it would take much longer.

Other People

Other people are very good memory aids as long as they don't become frustrated with your asking them for help remembering. This is a very good method for couples. For example, my wife often recalls certain things better than I do, such as routes. I can rely on her navigational skills and memory when I am driving in new places, which allows me to better concentrate on my driving. Of course, this often means that I take more time to learn the route if I have to travel it alone. As a matter of "family engineering," one member of a family often does the checkbook. Both members of the couple rely on the memory of that person to pay bills on time and to remember to balance the checkbook. Other family members may be called on to remember when to wash clothing, for example, or take out the garbage and recycling on the day the truck comes. There are many ways in which people who live with others use a team effort to remember critical aspects of what needs to be done.

The many methods reviewed above work very well to help us manage normal forgetting or compensate for the loss of efficiency in memory as we age. However, these techniques are also useful for anyone who had mild short-term memory loss, anterograde amnesia. The one caveat is that the technique must be mastered early in the course of memory loss. If you wait until you need the skill, you may not be able to learn it. The next two chapters will discuss the topic of clinical memory loss, specifically Mild Cognitive Impairment and Alzheimer's disease.

PART II

What Is

Memory Loss?

CHAPTER TEN

Mild Cognitive Impairment

So far, we have focused on challenges to memory that we all face and on general as well as specific ways to manage short-term memory and forgetting, enabling us to build stronger long-term memory in the areas of our choosing. The strategies and methods reviewed in earlier chapters will work for you whether you are struggling with demands of work or education, and whether you are still young or managing normal changes associated with growing older. This and the next chapter review the most common disorders of memory, Mild Cognitive Impairment and dementias. The major focus among the dementias is Alzheimer's disease because it is the one that seems to bring up the most fear for people and is also by far the most prevalent pathology that causes dementia.

The key to managing memory disorders is to catch them early and to develop and implement memory management strategies before your need them. Although the word "Alzheimer's" strikes fear in all of us, the actual disease unfolds over many years, probably decades, and progresses very slowly. This slow and progressive unfolding gives you the opportunity to control and manage your own future if you start early in the course of memory loss. Detecting the early signs of possible future progressive decline also gives researchers an opportunity to discover and develop techniques for slowing the course of the disease. Early detection of vulnerability to memory loss is more likely if one becomes familiar with the risk factors associated with conditions like Alzheimer's disease and is open to professional assessment and detection of clinically significant memory loss before it becomes more than just memory loss. Mild Cognitive Impairment appears to be the transition state for many who will later develop Alzheimer's disease and therefore will be our entry into the world of memory disorders.

An Overview of Mild Cognitive Impairment

Mild Cognitive Impairment is the earliest stage of memory loss. For some individuals, it may be a transitional state to Alzheimer's disease. One form of Mild Cognitive Impairment, the amnestic type, is demonstrated when a person suffers a greater than expected decline in memory performance on demanding memory tests when compared with his or her peers (see Table 1). Individuals who are affected by Mild Cognitive Impairment are not demented. Persons with Mild Cognitive Impairment of the amnestic type have poor short-term memory leading to difficulty with learning new information and recalling recent events. But they have good intellectual skills and are able to compensate for the memory loss well despite the inconvenience. If followed without treatment for six years, about 50 percent of individuals with this form of Mild Cognitive Impairment achieve a diagnosis of Alzheimer's disease (meaning that there are changes in mental functions in addition to decline of short-term memory).

Complicating the clinical picture of Mild Cognitive Impairment is the belief that there may be three subtypes of

TABLE 1

MILD COGNITIVE IMPAIRMENT OF THE AMNESTIC TYPE

Diagnostic Criteria for Mild Cognitive Impairment of the amnestic type:

— Memory complaint
— Intellectual functions are consistent with personal history
— Self-care is normal
— Short-term memory impairment on formal memory testing for age and education
— Not demented
— Speed of mental operations is slower than expected
— Mental flexibility is reduced

Some facts about Mild Cognitive Impairment of the amnestic type:

— Converts to Alzheimer's disease at rate of 10–15 percent per year (normal conversion rate without Mild Cognitive Impairment is 1–2 percent per year)
— 50 percent convert within 6 years, if untreated
— May convert more rapidly as age advances
— May exist in as many as 20 percent of those who are older than 75
— May be transition state for Alzheimer's disease
— No differences between sexes

Mild Cognitive Impairment. First, there is an amnestic type as described above and in Table 1. Second, there is a form of Mild Cognitive Impairment in which the person afflicted has adequate memory but displays a decline within a domain of mental function other than memory. For example, the afflicted person may display impairment in judgment, changes in personality, or decline in reasoning but have a good short-term memory. One client of mine who fit this subtype believed that he had won the Publisher's Clearinghouse Sweepstakes prize despite having a good short- and long-term memory. He even bought airplane tickets to go to another state to pick up his believed winnings. He did not win but was never persuaded otherwise. Third, there is a mixed type of Mild Cognitive Impairment in which there are multiple small changes in mental functions including remembering, decision making, and judgment.

Characteristics of Mild Cognitive Impairment

Formal criteria for the diagnosis of the amnestic form of Mild Cognitive Impairment are evolving, but we can consider the following as a working definition. First, there must be a complaint about short-term memory. Second, the short-term memory loss should be corroborated by an informant such as a spouse or other family member or close friend. However, I have evaluated many persons over the years who were rightly concerned about their own short-term memory despite the lack of concern by others including their spouse. It is often difficult to differentiate simple "senior moments" from actual mild short-term memory loss. Indeed, during the early stages of memory decline, we are often the best judges of our own weaknesses. If you have a feeling that your short-term memory is not right (or you are having failures in skills that you feel should work better, such as working with computer programs), it is important to seek an evaluation by someone trained in memory testing.

The third criteria in our working definition of the amnestic type of Mild Cognitive Impairment is that formal testing of the person reveals good intellectual ability consistent with his or her life history and accomplishments. Fourth, the person with the amnestic type of Mild Cognitive Impairment clearly can care for all personal needs without assistance or prompting. Fifth, the individual is not demented. This means the person can independently carry out all social, recreational, vocational, and avocational functions. One of the most startling professional lessons that I have learned is that you cannot identify those with Mild Cognitive Impairment by talking with them, by doing a brief mental state exam, or even by doing a thorough clinical interview. They pass all of these tests with flying colors.

The Importance of Early Detection of Mild Cognitive Impairment

The current interest in Mild Cognitive Impairment reflects our understanding of the need to detect Alzheimer's disease in its earliest stages. This is also true for conditions such as vascular dementia, Lewy body dementia, frontotemporal dementia, primary progressive aphasia, or other progressive conditions that may first be detected as Mild Cognitive Impairment. One of the most critical aspects of managing short-term memory loss is the need to establish compensation strategies before they are needed. Many clients have assured me that they will learn the skill (for example, of using a personal calendar) or make the appropriate change (such as stopping driving) when they need to. But this is exactly the rub for short-term memory loss: as memory loss progresses, you lose awareness of your mistakes. I had a client who had five documented accidents in her car in the previous month but thought she had a perfect driving record because she could not recall any of the incidents. Despite the intuitive belief that we should become less convinced of our convictions as memory loss increases, people who forget they forget often are more convinced of the reliability of their memory. This is why it is essential to learn to use external memory supports at the first signs of memory decline.

The habits you build today protect you tomorrow. Those who have Mild Cognitive Impairment need to establish their future plan, or "safety net," immediately in case there is further decline over time. The safety net should involve important family members and/or friends. Specific elements of this planning will be discussed in chapter 13. A person with Mild Cognitive Impairment has the capacity to comprehend and master strategies, such as those discussed in earlier chapters, to manage short-term memory loss. However, self-management becomes increasingly difficult to master as memory decline progresses and forgetting that you forget progresses. Thus, as short-term memory declines, a person is increasingly reliant on the routines, memory aids, and skills that he or she already has. At some point in the progression of Alzheimer's disease, new learning becomes nearly impossible. Furthermore, as short-term memory declines in Alzheimer's disease, other mental skills increasingly decay as well, including insight, planning, judgment, and reasoning. The bottom line here is to act early. Don't be afraid of Mild Cognitive Impairment. It is the opportunity to take control of your future.

A multitude of studies are under way to better determine the underlying changes in brain function/anatomy and cognition that occur within Mild Cognitive Impairment. Additionally, numerous studies are being done to determine which treatments can slow the "conversion" of Mild Cognitive Impairment to Alzheimer's disease. Trials include use of agents such as Aricept and Exelon in addition to vitamin E, anti-inflammatory agents, and Ginkgo biloba. There are also an increasing number of support groups and workshops to help persons with Mild Cognitive Impairment gain better control over their future.

How Do Professionals Detect Mild Cognitive Impairment?

Formal memory testing using tests like the California Verbal Learning Test or the Wechsler Memory Scale are the "gold standard" for early detection of both Mild Cognitive Impairment and Alzheimer's disease. Whatever memory test is given should evaluate both immediate and delayed recall and should be challenging. A thorough evaluation should assess not only memory but also other mental operations such as intelligence, reasoning, attention, constructive skills, and language. Formal testing can be used for monitoring the course of and response to treatments in those with Mild Cognitive Impairment as well as those with Alzheimer's disease or other progressive conditions.

Additionally, imaging studies involving use of structural Magnetic Resonance Imaging (MRI), Positron Emission Tomography (PET), and Single-Photon Emission Computed Tomography (SPECT)—especially serial volumetric MRIs and topographic detection—are receiving a great deal of attention as methods for early detection of Alzheimer's disease. Finally, longitudinal studies suggest that apolipoprotein E4 status may be predictive of those with Mild Cognitive Impairment who will later achieve a diagnosis of Alzheimer's disease as well as those who may progress more rapidly. This is a very intense area of research, clinical studies, and interventions.

Mild Cognitive Impairment as a Possible Transitional State for Alzheimer's Disease

Mild Cognitive Impairment may be a transitional condition between normal mental functioning and Alzheimer's disease. Alzheimer's disease is chronic and starts off in a very mild form. You do not suddenly wake up with Alzheimer's disease out of nowhere. Noticeable mental decline appears at least two to four years before a diagnosis of dementia can be made, and a "pre-clinical state" characterized by very mild deficits may extend for as many as 10 years before the disease can be clearly diagnosed. A decline in short-term memory (the kind of memory needed for development of new learning) is especially predictive of Alzheimer's disease (see Table 4 for a more complete listing of criteria for Alzheimer's disease).

At some point in the natural history of a case of Alzheimer's disease, there appears to be a point at which there is a more rapid decline in skills. This is the time when most seek medical diagnosis and treatment. I can do much more for those who come to me with Mild Cognitive Impairment than I can for those who already clearly have Alzheimer's disease. That is why it is essential that you not put off a professional consultation if you are concerned about your memory.

Signs of Possible Mild Cognitive Impairment to Watch For

At the earliest onset of Mild Cognitive Impairment, a person probably has a growing awareness that something is wrong, but friends and relatives are likely to suggest that the symptoms are the same as we all experience as we age, simply "senior moments." In addition to concerns about short-term memory, the person may also exhibit changes in behavior (such as depression or unusual irritability) that are often inexplicable at the time. One of my clients who detected a problem at a very early stage first became concerned that something was wrong with her when she was driving back to her home from a visit with her daughter. She had driven this same route of about 15 miles hundreds of times before, but on the occasion that caught her attention, she suddenly could not recall how to get home. She was clever and stopped at a restaurant to have coffee. After a short time, she recalled the route she needed to take. She was also clever in that she called for an assessment the following day. Changes, such as those described in Table 2, may go on for many years before an individual seeks a diagnosis. But the earlier we seek help, the more that can be done to help us manage the changes.

TABLE 2

CHANGES THAT MAY BE SIGNS OF MILD COGNITIVE IMPAIRMENT*

Mental Changes

— Concerns about your short-term memory

— Inability to follow through on projects

— Difficulty following thoughts through

— Difficulty with work

— Inability to hold onto a thought or an idea

— Gaps in logic that cannot be closed no matter how often others explain

Behavioral Changes

— Onset of depression

— Outbursts of irrational rage

— Intense suspicion and fear of others

— Hostile responses for no apparent reason

— Unbelievable stories of bad things done by others

— Sudden onset of drinking in a person who does not drink

*Adapted from Gray-Davidson, 1999

CHAPTER ELEVEN

Alzheimer's Disease and Dementia

Knowing that you have cancer tells you only the most general information about your condition, that you may have a serious and sometimes fatal illness. There are many different kinds of cancer: lung, prostate, breast, bone, pancreatic, basal cell, melanoma, glioma, meningioma, and so on. Each cancer has unique properties, course, prognosis, and treatment. One of the most frequent misunderstandings that I have encountered in my career as a memory specialist is based on a misconception about the term "dementia," which many don't understand is actually a general term like "cancer" for a number of kinds of disorders. Many clients have expressed relief because they have been told by someone, sometimes a professional, that they have "dementia" and therefore do not have Alzheimer's disease. I have also had clients who were told by professionals that they are "too old" to get Alzheimer's disease. These statements stem from a confusion of terminology. The terms "cancer" and "dementia" both represent superordinate categories that subsume many specific disorders, each with a unique cause and prognosis. As with cancer, there are many types or causes/etiologies of dementia. For example, causes of dementia may include closed head injury, stroke, Pick's disease, Lewy body disease, viruses, Parkinson's disease, and AIDS. Alzheimer's disease is the most frequent cause of dementia. More than half of all cases of dementia are a result of the plaques and tangles that are believed to be the pathology underlying Alzheimer's disease.

Dementia is a syndrome (constellation of signs and features) that requires systematic evaluation to determine the cause. Alzheimer's disease is a specific form of dementia that is caused by plaques and tangles in the neurons of the brain. Vascular dementia is a specific form of dementia that is caused by multiple small strokes. The former typically comes on slowly over years whereas the latter often comes on in a series of sudden changes or steps, although this distinction is not foolproof. Diffuse Lewy body (the name of a physician who identified these features in the brain) disease is a dementia that is caused by the pathologic changes in brain structure known as Lewy bodies. These and other specific names of dementias refer to the cause of the changes in neurons in the brain. Most simply, dementia is an often progressive, adult-onset deterioration of mental and adaptive functions that interferes with one's ability to live independently.

Definitions and Types of Dementia

There are two general technical sets of criteria used by professionals to define/diagnose dementia. These are drawn from professional sources such as the *International Classification of Disease* (ICD) and the *Diagnostic and Statistical Manual IV-TR* (DSM IV-TR) of the American Psychiatric Association. The more general definition for dementia requires that a person exhibit a persistent decline in at least three of five major mental domains. These domains include language (difficulty with expressing oneself with words, difficulty comprehending language), memory (difficulty learning new information or skills, recalling past information), visuospatial and visuoconstructive abilities (problems with navigation or route finding, difficulty with drawing), executive functions (deficits in judgment, reasoning, abstraction), praxis (difficulty dressing, using utensils to eat), and/or personality (becoming more passive or more irritable).

A more restrictive definition (see Table 3) requires impaired short-term memory accompanied by decline in at least one other mental domain that impairs occupational, social, or interpersonal functioning. The essential difference between these

TABLE 3

COMMONLY USED CRITERIA FOR DIAGNOSIS OF DEMENTIA

Impaired recent memory AND one or more of the following:

— Difficulty with reasoning

— Disorientation

— Difficulty with language

— Poor concentration

— Difficulty with spatial relationships

— Poor judgment

— Personality changes

— Changes in sexuality

— Delusional thinking

— Diminished coordination

— Diminished or lost sense of taste or smell

— Lower IQ

definitions is that the latter restricts the term to disorders that include memory loss, such as Alzheimer's disease, whereas the former does not make memory loss necessary for diagnosis.

Alzheimer's disease is the model for the second definition and has gained so much attention because it is clearly the main cause of dementia as we age. Approximately 56 percent of cases of dementia are caused be the plaques and tangles of Alzheimer's disease. About 14 percent of the remaining cases are a result of vascular processes whereas 10 percent are caused by Parkinson's disease and/or Lewy body disease. Finally, 8 percent of dementias are caused by frontotemporal diseases, and the remaining 12 percent are caused by either multiple factors or other causes. The projected number of persons who will develop Alzheimer's disease over the course of the next 50 years is staggering. Estimates suggest that there were 4 million cases of Alzheimer's disease in 2000. By 2010 the number of cases will grow to 5.9 million, and by 2050 estimates suggest that there will be 16 million cases of Alzheimer's disease in the United States. Table 4 presents a listing of several forms of dementia. Each is believed to have a different underlying cause, despite the fact that the external manifestations can be very similar. Keep in mind that real life is never as simple as our schemas. Many dementias are of mixed causes.

Diagnosing Dementia

The process of diagnosing a dementia, such as Alzheimer's disease, may take several years. The beginning of the disease is often subtle and variable in its time course as well as in symptoms. Many persons who will later develop Alzheimer's disease are first diagnosed with depression. There is no specific threshold for calling a decline in abilities a dementia or for changing the diagnosis from Mild Cognitive Impairment to Alzheimer's disease. Diagnosis is a complex clinical judgment. In Alzheimer's

---

TABLE 4

MAJOR TYPES OF DEMENTIAS

— Alzheimer's disease
— Pick's disease
— Frontotemporal dementia
— Vascular dementia
    Lacunar state
    Binswanger's disease
— Lewy body disease
— Parkinson's dementia
— Supranuclear palsy
— Huntington's disease
— Infections
    General paresis
    Slow virus infections
    Creutzfeldt-Jacob disease
— Hydrocephalis
— Demylenating diseases
— HIV encephalopathy
— Semantic dementia
— Dementia resulting from head injury
— Neoplastic disease

---

disease there may be a several-year period of memory loss and sometimes language loss that begins with Mild Cognitive Impairment, which itself may have a several-year course. Even the early stages of Alzheimer's disease may not be severe enough to label the disease a dementia. Evaluation and ultimate diagnosis is a process that may require complex and repeated assessment over time.

Risk Factors for Alzheimer's Disease

There are currently about 13.5 million cases of Alzheimer's disease in developed countries. If the prevalence rate remains as it is today, there will be 36.7 million cases by 2050, 16 million of those in the United States. If we can develop a medication that slows the progress of the disease by five years, we can cut the prevalence in half, to about 8 million cases in the United States by 2050. Epidemiological studies suggest that the greatest risk factor for developing Alzheimer's disease is older age. Persons who live to be between 85 and 90 have nearly a 50 percent chance of developing Alzheimer's disease, and those living to be 95 have about a 60 percent chance of developing Alzheimer's disease. Add to this the fact that about 50 to 60 percent of persons with short-term memory loss but otherwise intact mental skills (that is, with Mild Cognitive Impairment) will be diagnosed with Alzheimer's disease after about five years if no treatments are provided. Clearly, the risk is greatest for those who are aging and who already experience significant short-term memory loss when compared with their peers. But note that the outcome is not 100 percent. Neither aging nor short-term memory loss is a sentence for eventually having Alzheimer's disease.

There are several other risk factors that add vulnerability for development of Alzheimer's disease, but none is as strongly associated with the disease as is age or short-term memory loss. A primary relative (parent or sibling) with Alzheimer's disease increases the risk of developing this disease, but the relationship of genetics and Alzheimer's disease is complex. A majority of the persons who have come to me for assessment do not have a primary relative with Alzheimer's disease. One of the patients whom I assessed was a terrified woman in her 60s. Her identical twin was in a nursing home with Alzheimer's disease. Fortunately, she had an excellent memory and mental skills.

Despite this, the risk is increased with multiple family members with memory loss late in life. For example, a physician in his 70s asked for assessment of his memory because he was one of seven children in his family, and all of his siblings had a diagnosis of Alzheimer's disease. (A small number of families have a dramatic risk of developing Alzheimer's disease usually relatively early in their life.) The assessment showed that he had Mild Cognitive Impairment. Still, family history is far less than perfect in predicting Alzheimer's disease and has less impact on risk than do age and Mild Cognitive Impairment.

Another genetic factor to be considered is the presence of apolipoprotein E4 (a gene that modulates cholesterol metabolism and may also have a role in cardiovascular disease). There are three forms of a gene known as apolipoprotein (coded on chromosome 19) known as E2, E3, and E4. You receive one of these genes from each parent leading to combinations such as E2 - E2, E2 - E4, etc. We now know that anyone with an E4 is at somewhat higher risk of developing Alzheimer's disease, and anyone with an E2 is less likely to develop Alzheimer's disease. Again, the relationship is complicated and not diagnostic in that there are many with E4 who do not develop Alzheimer's disease and some with E2 who do.

Other risk factors for developing Alzheimer's disease include having sustained a closed head injury at some earlier time in your life. I have seen a number of persons in their 60s and 70s whose first concerns began after what appeared to be a mild head trauma. However, I have also seen a number of persons with past history of head trauma who did not develop Alzheimer's disease. Apolipoprotein E4 may also play a role in this situation. A history of depression in later life is also associated with the development of Alzheimer's disease. Many who have depression have changes in their brains as determined by imaging studies such as the MRI, and this relationship is currently under careful evaluation in many clinics.

Women are slightly more likely to develop Alzheimer's disease than are men, but this advantage for men is small and may disappear for those who are older than 85. Also, persons with lower educational attainment (probably having less than a ninth-grade education) are more vulnerable. The more interesting question here may be the association of "brightness" with Alzheimer's disease. Do those who start out brighter have more mental reserve and therefore more ability to fend off the impact of Alzheimer's disease longer? Can mental stimulation increase mental reserve in all of us? This may be an area where we can exercise some control by how we spend our time earlier in life.

Cardiovascular disease also presents increased vulnerability to developing Alzheimer's disease. This again may be related to the apolipoprotein gene type. Unlike the factors discussed earlier, this clearly implies that lifestyle may influence the onset of Alzheimer's disease. This is an area where we have some control. Therefore, it is critical to manage hypertension (especially systolic hypertension), cholesterol, diabetes, and lifestyle (by not smoking, limiting alcohol consumption to two drinks per day, exercising, and eating well) to prevent and/or minimize cardiovascular disease and to protect our brain. This is especially important given the findings that those with the greatest mental impairment appear to have both the plaques and tangles of Alzheimer's disease and the small strokes that represent the damage from cardiovascular disease.

Knowing the risk factors provides control. If you have several risk factors, you should assess the choices you are making about your lifestyle and plan ahead. Consider seeking guidance from a memory expert should you experience concerns about either your memory or your mental skills. Knowing the risk factors also helps researchers identify those who are more vulnerable and devise tests of substances (medications, vitamins, herbs) and lifestyle changes that can potentially slow or prevent the progression of Alzheimer's disease. The discovery of a large group of persons with Mild Cognitive Impairment, also known as isolated anterograde amnesia, has provided an opportunity to gain some control over the course of memory loss and Alzheimer's disease. It allows predication of high risk individuals for early management and for clinical trials to determine what works and what doesn't work to slow or prevent progression.

A Metric for Understanding and Tracking the Changes in Alzheimer's Disease

To better understand the complex nature of the changes that may occur during Alzheimer's disease, let's review the stages of the Global Deterioration Scale (devised by Reisberg, Ferris, de Leon, and Crook in 1982). The Global Deterioration Scale is a seven-point rating scale for staging the magnitude of changes in mental and functional capacity that begins with forgetfulness and ends in severe Alzheimer's disease. The changes represented by this scale are very gross generalizations that allow rough judgments to be made of progression of the disease, but specific movement through the stages is inexact. However, this scale helps us view the natural history of Alzheimer's disease which may take anywhere from 3 to 20 years after diagnosis.

NORMAL

The first stage in this scale is the stage we all aspire to remain in for the duration of our life. This stage includes the changes in mental efficiency that are associated with normal aging. In this stage, there are no complaints of memory loss by self or others. Furthermore, there is no objective evidence of memory loss from either clinical interview or objective assessment.

FORGETFULNESS

In the second stage, called "Forgetfulness" a person presents with subjective complaints about short-term memory loss but does not appear to show memory loss either during casual observation or during a careful clinical interview. Forgetful persons do well on screening tests and can only be identified through well-constructed memory testing. Forgetfulness may be the earliest presentation of the amnestic variant of Mild Cognitive Impairment, and individuals in this stage are appropriately concerned about changes in their memory. Others may justify these changes as "senior moments," but in reality the person is experiencing real changes. The instances of forgetting are often exaggerations of normal memory failures, such as forgetting where things are placed or forgetting names that one knows well. These are things we all do occasionally. We do not know how long this stage may last.

CONFUSIONAL STATES

The next two stages are known as the "Early Confusional State" and the "Late Confusional State," respectively. A person in the Early Confusional State may get lost when traveling in familiar locations. Also, spouses or friends may become concerned about deficits in skills and/or in word and name finding. The person with memory loss may not be as aware as are others of the changes, but typical clinical interviews and screening tests may still not be able to detect the changes in memory. As the disease progresses into a Late Confusional State, there is a decline in knowledge of current and recent events. There is a loss in ability to travel independently and to handle finances. Deficits are now clear in interview and screening tests. The person may be quite befuddled but can usually survive on his or her own.

During the progression of confusional states, there are progressive changes in communication that are typical of the early stages of Alzheimer's disease. My cat functions very well in her world despite the fact that she cannot speak a human word. But human beings are bound by language. Although we all know much more than we can say, alterations in language and communication brought on by the progression of Alzheimer's disease profoundly affect both the person with disease and the receivers of the communication.

We all spend more time searching for words as we age. However, in Alzheimer's disease the problem goes beyond normal frustrations of word finding. As Alzheimer's disease progresses, vocabulary shrinks and simpler, more common words are often substituted for specific terms. In other words, a person with Alzheimer's disease is more likely to refer to "stuff" or "thing" rather than to say "fork" or "cat." The "clock" becomes "the thing that tells time" as function words (called circumlocutions) replace nouns. These changes in language lead the afflicted person to become increasingly quiet especially in lengthier conversations or in groups as they cannot find words fast enough to keep up with the flow of conversation. Also contributing to increased quietness is the growing struggle caused by forgetting what has just been said either by oneself or by others.

The cohesiveness of speech in a person in the early stages of Alzheimer's disease begins to deteriorate, and pronouns are overused. A reduction of executive functions (abstraction, reasoning) makes jokes and sarcasm confusing. Reading comprehension declines, and in combination with increased short-term memory loss, the person becomes less interested in reading. Despite these changes, the mechanics of writing tend to be good. However, the combination of memory loss and poor initiation makes writing increasingly difficult. This results in a deterioration of the ability to correspond, make notes for oneself, and use e-mail.

EARLY DEMENTIA STAGE

The next stage in the Global Deterioration Scale is called the "Early Dementia Stage" and may last five years. People in this stage cannot recall major personal information such as their phone number or address of many years. They often forget the names of their grandchildren or the name of the high school or college from which they graduated. There is often some disorientation to time (such as claiming that the current year is 2000 or missing the month) or to place (reporting that they are in Michigan when they are in Florida or not being able to recall the town in which they currently reside). Persons in the Early Dementia Stage do not need assistance with personal care such as using the toilet or dressing, but they cannot survive without some assistance or a companion. During this stage a person can clearly do well with supervision and support from a spouse.

Language skills further erode during the Early Dementia Stage. Language is often reduced to the level of a five- to seven-year-old. Reading aloud is spared as are the mechanics of writing, but initiation and memory loss make it unlikely that these skills will be displayed unless prompted by others. A person in early dementia retains automatic and social phrases. However, individuals at this stage have less to say and use more words to communicate fewer ideas. The content of their speech is shorter and less complex. Hence, speech of a person in the Early Dementia Stage is labeled as "empty," making their conversations disjointed and difficult to follow.

Increasing memory loss and the struggle with self-monitoring (tracking what they have just said) causes those in this stage to frequently repeat ideas as if they are being said for the first time. As the disease progresses, comprehension of spoken and written language declines and interpretations become literal and concrete. For example, I asked a person during a memory screening to spell the word "world" backwards. She proceeded to turn her back to me and spelled "w-o-r-l-d." She then turned back to me and asked, "How did I do?" Communication for the person in the Early Dementia Stage becomes more dependent upon context, intonation, gestures, and behavior. In this stage, first languages are better retained than second languages. Often, prompting and modeling are better forms of communication than is speech. In short, Alzheimer's disease is accompanied by progressive aphasia making communication via speech to and by the person with Alzheimer's disease more and more difficult.

MIDDLE DEMENTIA STAGE

The last two stages are the ones that most of us fear. Indeed, these are the stages that underlay a recent headline in the *New York Times* (November 11, 2002): "More than death, many elderly fear dementia." These are the stages where disability rather than annoyance and inconvenience takes over. The earlier of the two last stages is called "Middle Dementia Stage." A person in this stage may not always know the name of his or her spouse or children. He or she will be unaware of recent events and experiences. This reflects the increasing toll of anterograde amnesia. His or her knowledge of the past becomes sketchy because there is a progressive erosion of remote memory (called retrograde amnesia). I recall my surprise when a woman whom I was interviewing had completely forgotten that she had a mastectomy a month earlier. A person in the Middle Dementia Stage will have increasing difficulty with personal care, such as knowing when to change clothing or how often or how to shower. Personality and emotional changes are also likely to occur in this stage (such as increased passivity or irritability), and the person needs considerable guidance and environmental support to engage even in pleasing activities.

LATE DEMENTIA STAGE

Finally, some are unfortunate enough to arrive at "Late Stage Dementia." In this stage all verbal skills are lost, and the person is largely mute and in need of total care. The brain has lost its ability to engage in the basic skills we all take for granted such as being able to walk, talk, and eat. Fortunately, most with Alzheimer's disease do not live to this stage.

The Montessori Model

The educational schema known as the Montessori method (named after its founder) has increasingly been applied to Alzheimer's disease. The Montessori model was originally formulated as an alternative to traditional childhood education. The model is based on human development and has the advantage that it is more practical than descriptive. It does not arise from a medical model and is not pathology based. Montessori principles can be applied to assist with the development of treatment programs for persons with dementia.

The basic rule of thumb for the Montessori model as applied to Alzheimer's disease is that as skills decline, they disappear in the reverse order of their initial appearance. In short, "first in, last out." Thus the first skills to decline are higher level skills such as giving lectures or writing books. As the disease progresses, skills involved in doing taxes or using the computer may break down. With further progression, the ability to travel independently or pick out appropriate clothes to wear deteriorates. It is only later in the progression of the disease that the ability to tend to personal needs and to use language regresses. Montessori principles guide the development and implementation of self-correcting activities that focus on participation and retained skills rather than on correctness. As the decline progresses, caregivers (intimates as well as professionals) need to arrange activities that are designed around automatic behaviors and environmental cues and do not require recall or memory. The idea is that production is more important than competence. This adds to rather than defeats self-esteem.

Whether you are more comfortable with a clinical model such as that reflected in the Global Deterioration Scale or an educational model such as that reflected in the Montessori model, it is clear that the changes that occur in the course of a progressive dementia require less use of talking and language and more use of demonstration, imitation, and prompting. There needs to be a shift from doing for to being with. This general approach to management of memory disorders increases self-esteem and self-respect. It suggests that we need to think in terms of adapting the environment to the person rather than adapting the person to the environment. We shall return to a discussion of these principles in chapter 13.

Evaluation for Alzheimer's Disease

The tools used to evaluate and diagnose Mild Cognitive Impairment and Alzheimer's disease have greatly improved over the past decade. The recommended evaluation consists of gathering a detailed history from the affected individual and a family member or companion who knows the person being evaluated well. The evaluation should contain a standardized mental status exam, a general neurological exam, and laboratory tests (chemistry, B12, thyroid, etc.). Neuroimaging studies such as a Magnetic Resonance Imaging (MRI) or Computerized Tomography (CT) scan are also recommended. Finally, a neuropsychological evaluation is recommended to provide a description of strengths and weaknesses, to provide a baseline for evaluation of treatments, and to monitor changes over time. A neuropsychological evaluation consists of a challenging and standardized memory test as well as an assessment of other mental skills such as intellectual ability, construction, language, and problem solving.

Many studies are under way to determine if there are accurate and reliable biological markers for Alzheimer's disease. So far, there are no clear biological markers. The most promising candidates are being studied through the use of serial volumetric MRI, measuring A-Beta amyloid in cerebrospinal fluid and measuring A-Beta-42 amyloid in plasma, and quantitative MRI. It does not appear that testing for apolipoprotein (the gene discussed in chapter 11) is very helpful at this time, from a clinical point of view.

In summary, it is in our own best interests to identify and treat Mild Cognitive Impairment early rather than waiting until it progresses into Alzheimer's disease. There is growing evidence that the use of cholinesterase inhibitors such as Aricept, Exelon, or Reminyl (discussed in the next chapter) slows the progression of Alzheimer's disease. Presumably, treatment of Mild Cognitive Impairment with one of these medications could delay the "conversion" to Alzheimer's disease. The best way to manage Alzheimer's disease is early detection and early planning. There are warning signs that should lead us to seek professional evaluation. If you notice any of the changes described in Table 5 in yourself or in others you care about, take action early.

TABLE 5

SIGNS OF POSSIBLE EARLY STAGE DEMENTIA*

Mental Changes

— Overall inability to function as well as before

— Memory loss affecting job performance

— Having difficulty performing a familiar task

— Forgetting simple words

— Using inappropriate words

— Getting lost in time or place

— Exercising poor judgment

— Having problems with abstract thinking (e.g., trouble adding numbers)

— Misplacing things and putting them in odd places (e.g., milk in the cupboard)

— Having problems dealing with household bills and documents

— Having domestic accidents

— Leaving appliances on

— Leaving pots burning on the stove

— Getting lost in the car or having a series of unaccounted for car accidents

— Being unable to account for the day's activities

— Showing inconsistency in memory or behavior

———————
*Adapted from Gray-Davidson, 1999

Table 5 continued on next page

TABLE 5 (continued)

SIGNS OF POSSIBLE EARLY STAGE DEMENTIA*

Behavioral Changes

— Displaying rapid mood changes for no obvious reason

— Displaying sudden or gradual dramatic changes in personality

— Losing initiative or interest in usual pursuits

— Deteriorating in appearance

— Making changes in grooming and dress

— Wearing slightly odd combinations of clothing

— Declining in personal hygiene

— Dropping old friendships and social patterns

— Becoming more dependent

— Avoiding contact with close family members

— Staying in bed for long periods without reason

— Telling stories about neighbors doing bad things

— Relating strange events

— Calling the police for no valid reason

— Having changes in sleep patterns

— Having little or no food in the refrigerator or cupboards

— Having spoiled or expired food in the refrigerator or cupboards

— Hoarding

— Displaying mood changes that seem to be unrelated to external events

---

*Adapted from Gray-Davidson, 1999

PART III

What Can You Do

to Protect

Yourself?

CHAPTER TWELVE

Managing Your Biology: *Medications, Supplements, and Foods*

Now that you better understand memory and its disorders, it's time to turn to ways to protect yourself. What can you control? You cannot control genes, family history, or the life you have already lived. But there are factors that you and I *can* control. The potentially controllable risk factors for developing memory loss are lifestyle, diet, and mental stimulation. Changes in lifestyle choices that you can make now may improve your odds of aging successfully.

Unfortunately, making these choices does not give any of us a guarantee. The studies currently available suggesting what to eat or what supplements to take are not always clear and are often contradictory. In this chapter, I have approached the task of recommending what to do as a consumer. In short, what would *I* want to know about medications, supplements, foods, and lifestyle for me or someone I love?

The treatment of memory loss has been so "medicalized" that many are waiting for cures for chronic and disabling diseases like Alzheimer's disease. Many await the "magic bullet" that will make cancers, heart disease, diabetes, and neurological disorders go away. This belief probably stems from the development of antibiotics that can cure bacterial infections (viral infections are another issue, as can be attested to by anyone who has had shingles) and immunizations for diseases like polio and smallpox.

However, as I search my memory for true cures for diseases during my lifetime, I find none. We did not find a cure for polio or for smallpox; rather, we found a way to keep them from developing in the first place. We were hopeful that the discovery of insulin would cure diabetes mellitus. It did not. Insulin clearly helps manage the disease and slow its progression, but replacement of insulin does not cure diabetes. The discovery of a way to increase dopamine in the brain (a chemical messenger that is deficient in those who develop Parkinson's disease) provided hope that we could cure Parkinson's disease. But again, this was not a cure. We can better manage Parkinson's disease with current dopamine-enhancing medications, but we have not cured this neurological disease. We cannot reliably cure cancers although modern treatments improve survival in many and cure cancers in some.

Given this history, why do we have such high hopes that a cure for Alzheimer's disease, a complex and progressive disease of the brain, will be found? We have medications that slow the progression of the disease in many and help with management of the disease. But if we rely only on medications, we fall short of what we can do to manage Alzheimer's disease. We must do much more.

The best models for understanding how to manage Mild Cognitive Impairment and Alzheimer's disease are found in our understanding of management of diabetes mellitus and Parkinson's disease. These diseases require us to detect vulnerability to the disease early and to manage lifestyle as well as medications if we acquire the disease. Early interventions with lifestyle are critical to manage later stages of these diseases and to modify their course, and management is a lifelong commitment. Similarly, there may be factors in early, middle, and later life that influence the course of many memory disorders. Early strategies require the modification of lifestyle and environment during development through early adulthood. Middle life strategies involve further lifestyle management as well as protection of the cardiovascular system and the brain. Finally, these strategies carry into later life and, hopefully, provide benefits whether or not it is our destiny to develop a dementia.

This and the next two chapters address factors that you can control or for which you can plan. Some of the factors discussed improve mental efficiency or reduce damage to the cerebrovascular system and therefore may help memory and mental functions in healthy adults. Others factors to be discussed have been shown to help memory and mental functions in those who are quite vulnerable to memory decline or already have memory or mental decline. Good memory hygiene calls for us to use the techniques discussed in the earlier chapters of the book to manage our memory throughout our life. Good memory hygiene also calls for us to attend to ways to improve our odds as we age and become vulnerable to disorders of memory, and to plan ahead for the inevitable changes in efficiency and possible decline that we hope will never happen to either us or to those we love. Creating a good safety net takes time and effort, but the benefits will be felt for years and decades to come.

Medications for Mild Cognitive Impairment and Dementias like Alzheimer's Disease

The first medication to be approved for the treatment of Alzheimer's disease was Cognex (tacrine). (Trade names are outside of parentheses and generic names are inside parentheses.) Cognex was the first medication from a class of drugs called cholinesterase inhibitors (see Table 6) that was introduced in the United States in the early 1990s as a treatment for Alzheimer's disease. This class of medications was developed based on the finding that a chemical messenger called acetyl-choline was deficient in the brains of persons with Alzheimer's disease. Similar to the logic for treating diabetes and Parkinson's disease, it was felt that replacement of this neurotransmitter would restore mental functions and memory in patients with Alzheimer's disease. Cholinesterase inhibitors like Cognex make more acetylcholine available by deactivating the enzyme in synapses (gaps between neurons) that deactivate acetylcholine once it has conveyed its message, thereby making more of acetylcholine available to compensate for the loss due to the disease.

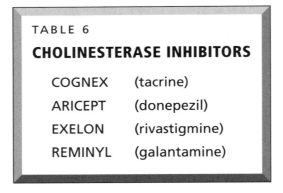

TABLE 6

CHOLINESTERASE INHIBITORS

COGNEX (tacrine)
ARICEPT (donepezil)
EXELON (rivastigmine)
REMINYL (galantamine)

The initial enthusiasm for Cognex was tempered by its side effects. Cognex produced changes in liver function in many who took this medication, so everyone on the medication needed to undergo frequent liver tests and, if there were changes in liver function, they had to stop treatment before per-manent damage was done. Cognex also produced a very high incidence of side effects (nausea, vomiting, diarrhea) that made it intolerable to a substantial proportion of those who took it. Finally, Cognex had to be taken four times a day, and building up to a therapeutic dose of Cognex was a long and complicated process that was more likely to produce side effects than a treatment response.

Fortunately, a second cholinesterase inhibitor, Aricept (donepezil), was approved by the FDA in 1996. Aricept does not have the incidence of side effects that Cognex does, and it does not cause liver toxicity. It is also easier to use as it is administered once a day rather than four times a day (as with Cognex), and there is only one increase in dose (from 5 to 10 mg) after four to six weeks on the medication. More recently, two newer cholinesterase inhibitors have been introduced into the market in the United States. Exelon (rivastimine) is similar to Aricept in action but must be taken twice a day. Higher doses of Exelon are more effective than lower doses, but these higher doses also produce more severe side effects. Reminyl (galantamine) was the last of these medications to be introduced. It also must be taken twice a day and has an incidence of side effects similar to that of Aricept.

The improvements from these medications are usually modest, and some recipients do not display any apparent effect of the medication. This leads some clients and their caregivers to wonder if the medication is doing them any good and to consider cessation of the medication, especially given the expense of these drugs. However, those who have stopped taking the medication have often shown a dramatic drop in functioning, and reinstating the medication does not reverse the changes to the level they would have been if they had kept taking the medication all along. Therefore, once a cholinesterase inhibitor has been started, it must be taken continuously unless there are intolerable side effects or a medical condition that conflicts with use of the drug.

Treatment Effects of Cholinesterase Inhibitors

Cholinesterase inhibitors do not cure or prevent Alzheimer's disease. They address only one of many possible neurochemical changes found in Alzheimer's disease, which is decreased cholinergic activity. They do not return the user to "normal" mental or memory functioning. Rather, these medications improve cognitive functions in some and may preserve ability to do self care for a longer time when compared to placebo.

I have not been impressed with changes in memory with the use of these medications. Rather, it appears that these medications often improve initiative and skills that we need to better manage memory, preserve mental and personal care, and facilitate interactions with the world around those who are experiencing mental decline. For example, treatment may lead one to be more likely to enter into a conversation or to pick up and read a magazine. Furthermore, when persons on one of these medications are observed over the course of a year, they score higher on cognitive tests and on tests of instrumental activities (using the telephone, handling mail, preparing food) and basic activities (dressing, eating, using the toilet) of daily living than those given a placebo. Cholinesterase inhibitors also reduce the time caregivers need to provide care and may reduce problematic behaviors such as delusions, agitation, anxiety, and disinhibition.

As an example, Marilyn Truscott was diagnosed with Alzheimer's disease in the late 1990s. After being placed on a cholinesterase inhibitor, she writes: "Thank heaven for the new Alzheimer medications now available. I could hold on to thoughts and words better when I read them or heard them spoken. I could understand information and instructions better. I had vastly more mental stamina to carry out activities and social conversations. My brain wouldn't tire out so quickly" (Truscott, 2003, p. 12).

In short, these medications appear to slow the decline in mental skills and behavior seen in persons with Alzheimer's disease when compared to those who are treated with a placebo. Early initiation of treatment with a cholinesterase inhibitor is associated with greater benefits when compared with later initiation. Furthermore, a recent clinical trial of these medications demonstrated improvement of mental functioning in persons with Mild Cognitive Impairment, and treatment with Aricept improved judgments made by airline pilots who had normal memory and mental abilities in a flight simulator. Presumably, if the medication were used earlier in the course of mental decline in Alzheimer's disease, or, better yet, if it were begun while the person was in the stage of Mild Cognitive Impairment, treatment would slow progression and improve the quality of life when compared to those who do not take one of these medications.

Side Effects of Cholinesterase Inhibitors

The most common side effects of cholinesterase inhibitors are fatigue, diarrhea, nausea, vomiting, anorexia (loss of appetite and weight), muscle cramps, dizziness, and rhinitis (inflammation of the nasal mucosa leading to congestions and increased secretion of mucus). These medications can also induce vivid dreams and/or nightmares and induce fainting in some. Side effects vary with dose. That is, the higher the dose, the greater incidence of side effects, and side effects are more likely to occur when the dose of the medication is increased. The incidences of side effects for the three cholinesterase inhibitors used today are Aricept 5-10 percent, Reminyl 5-40 percent, and Exelon 10-50 percent. These data suggest that Aricept and Reminyl are the best tolerated of the medications available in this class.

Although few studies have compared these agents against the other cholinesterase inhibitors, there appears to be no clinically significant advantage of any of the drugs. Therefore, side effect profile and ease of use are the most important determinants of which medication to use. If someone is intolerant of one of the medications, another can be tried and sometimes may be well tolerated. It is also important to note that cholinesterase inhibitors are effective for both Alzheimer's and vascular dementias and may have benefits for those with other forms of dementia such as Lewy body disease.

Namenda (Memantine)

Namenda (memantine) is a new drug in a different class of medication that has been used in Germany to treat Alzheimer's disease for more than a decade. It affects a different neurotransmitter system (glutamate is an excitatory neurotransmitter whose effect is believed to be reduced in the brain by memantine through its action of blocking the N-methyl-D-aspartate or NMDA receptors) and has been used for persons with moderate to severe Alzheimer's disease as well as in patients with pain syndromes because it also has an analgesic action. Recent trials suggest that Aricept and Namenda work together to improve the functioning of persons with severe Alzheimer's disease. Namenda has been approved by the FDA for release in the United States to become available in early 2004.

Vitamin E

There is evidence that supplementation of vitamin E may slow Alzheimer's disease. These results are from a major clinical study demonstrating that administration of a high dose of Vitamin E (1,000 international units (IU) two times per day) slowed the progression of Alzheimer's disease. Persons already afflicted by Alzheimer's disease who were treated with Vitamin E took several months longer to decline to the point where they needed placement in a skilled nursing facility and did not die as soon as those in the study who received the placebo. The same effect was also found with selegiline (trade names for selegiline are Eldepryl and Desprenyl). However, vitamin E is preferred clinically as it has fewer side effects and is cheaper than selegiline. A recent study demonstrated that high intake of vitamin E via diet correlated with higher mental function in men and women between the ages of 65 and 100 without Alzheimer's disease when compared to those who did not ingest foods high in vitamin E content. The same researchers showed a similar effect in persons with diagnosed Alzheimer's disease. These findings have led many clinicians to recommend that Alzheimer's disease be treated with a cholinesterase inhibitor and a high dose of vitamin E. There are currently clinical trails under way to determine if use of vitamin E slows the "progression" of Mild Cognitive Impairment into Alzheimer's disease. But as is the case with all substances that one ingests or otherwise administers, there is a cost to the use of vitamin E at the doses recommended.

Taking vitamin E, especially at high doses, may produce serious side effects. Vitamin E can potentiate anticoagulants such as aspirin or Coumadin, and it may promote bruising. Although Vitamin E may improve immune function in lower doses, it may suppress immune function when taken at doses above 1500 IUs. A recent study of institutionalized elderly in the Netherlands suggested that use of vitamin E was correlated with slower resolution of acute respiratory tract infections as well as the production of more symptoms per episode. Supplementation with vitamin E did not affect the incidence of the infections or the severity of symptoms experienced by those who developed the respiratory infection. Given the risks of using high doses of Vitamin E, some physicians recommend that only those with clear Alzheimer's disease should take 2,000 IUs, and that others, such as those with Mild Cognitive Impairment, should not take doses above 1500 IUs. Higher doses of vitamin E than those recommended in the standard Recommended Daily (or Dietary) Allowance (RDA) should not be taken without supervision of a physician.

There is more to the story of vitamin E as an antioxidant therapy. Presumably, vitamin E is administered to those with Alzheimer's disease to modify lipoproteins, which are thought pathogenic to the disease. However, Vitamin E alone does not curtail oxidation of lipoproteins in cerebrospinal fluid (an index of activity of substances in the central nervous system). Supplementation of vitamin E with vitamin C does curtail oxidation of lipoproteins. Retrospective studies suggest persons taking vitamin E and C together have better memory performance and less mental decline than those who take either vitamin alone. Therefore, it may be advisable to take vitamin E and vitamin C together. So far, it is not clear what the optimal dose of vitamin C is, but some physicians seem to favor 500 mg per day.

Vitamin B

Another vitamin to consider is vitamin B. There are a number of B vitamins, but it appears that folate (or folic acid) and vitamin B12 may be important for those trying to protect memory. These vitamins are critical in the formation of RNA and DNA, the building blocks of cells, including neurons. One step in the synthesis of RNA and DNA is the conversion of an amino acid named homocysteine into an amino acid named methionine. Vitamin B12 and folate enable this conversion, and when they are low, homocysteine builds up. Increased plasma concentrations of homocysteine are associated with increased risk of cardiovascular disease and progression of dementia. Low levels of vitamin B12 are associated with anemia, memory loss, and nerve damage. Low levels of folate are associated with cardiovascular disease. Supplementation of these vitamins may also slow mental decline, and dietary folate has been shown to cut the risk of stroke.

Given these relationships, many physicians are including an evaluation of concentration of homocysteine in blood tests during physicals. This may be even more critical for persons with Alzheimer's or vascular disease or those who may be vulnerable to these conditions. Some physicians recommend consumption of 1.0 micrograms of vitamin B12 and 400 micrograms of folate per day.

Other Antioxidants

There are many antioxidants in addition to vitamins E and C that may be protective of memory and mental function. These may also slow the progression of Mild Cognitive Impairment and/or Alzheimer's and vascular disease. For example, lycopene is an antioxidant found in tomatoes. Catechin is an antioxidant found in green and black teas. Tumeric is an antioxidant found in curry powder and mustards (especially the yellow mustard). Vitamin E can be increased in our diet by eating nuts and oils. Vitamin C and other antioxidants can be ingested in foods such as strawberries, blueberries, melons, spinach, Brussels sprouts, and tomato juice. One cup of orange juice per day provides 100 percent of the RDA of vitamin C for men and for women. The bottom line appears to be that we may do ourselves and our memory good by eating our fruits and vegetables.

Ginkgo biloba is a derivative of an Asiatic tree leaf. Ginkgo has antioxidant properties and also may have the ability to improve cerebral circulation. Ginkgo is currently available as a treatment for dementia in Germany and is available in the United States as an herbal supplement. A 1997 study in the United States suggested a modest improvement in people with dementia who took Ginkgo biloba. There are several trials of

Ginkgo currently under way with individuals who already have memory impairment as well as those with Mild Cognitive Impairment. The evidence that Ginkgo has a beneficial action has not always been demonstrated. For example, a recent study indicated that supplementation with 40 mg of Ginkgo biloba three times per day for six weeks in healthy older adults did not improve their learning, memory, or attention when compared to treatment with a placebo. Therefore, treatment with Ginkgo may not be of benefit to healthy older adults with normal memory and mental functions.

Despite some failures to find treatment effects for Ginkgo, millions of Americans take this herb in the hope that Ginkgo will either improve their memory or treat or delay the onset of Alzheimer's disease. Interestingly, the brands of Ginkgo biloba sold in the United States show considerable variation in quality and consistency. A study by the World Health Organization demonstrated that few of the brands it tested actually contained Ginkgo at the dose labeled on the bottles. As with many other substances, Ginkgo has potential side effects including nausea, heartburn, headache, dizziness, excessive bleeding or bruising, and low blood pressure. Because of its anticoagulant properties, Ginkgo may potentiate the effects of blood thinning drugs such as aspirin and Coumadin. There are also claims of an interaction of Ginkgo with caffeine that can lead to the formation of blood clots in the brain. Furthermore, Ginkgo can influence the secretion of insulin, making it risky for diabetics. Just because something is labeled "natural" or considered a food supplement does not mean that it is harmless. If you feel that you want to take Ginkgo, or other supplements, consult with your physician.

Omega-3 Fatty Acids

High caloric and high fat content in the diet may be a risk factor for Alzheimer's disease. Conversely, a diet containing low

levels of fat and cholesterol has been associated with a lower
risk of mental decline. High fat intake in midlife has been associated with an increased risk of later development of Alzheimer's
disease. These and similar findings have led to the suggestion
that a low fat, low cholesterol diet may be protective of memory
and mental functions. But the story on fats is complicated.
Omega-3 fatty acids (docosahexaenic acid or DHA) may
increase acetylcholine, and consumption of omega-3–rich fish
oil may boost mood and memory. Omega-3 fatty acids are
referred to as the "good fats" whereas omega-6 fatty acids
(found in steaks and other animal fats) are referred to as the
"bad fats." Given this distinction, it may be farsighted to eat at
least two servings a week of fish such as tuna, salmon, swordfish,
sole, and cod. The take-away story is to supplement your fruits
and vegetables with fish rich in omega-3 fatty acids as another
possible way to reduce your vulnerability to memory and mental
decline.

Statins

Further suggesting the need to regulate fat and cholesterol
intake is the recent epidemiologic finding of a decreased prevalence of Alzheimer's disease associated with the use of medications known as statins. Statins are widely used to reduce high
cholesterol (hypercholesterolemia). Statins include the medications Zocor, Lipitor, and Pravachol. Whether the benefit from
taking statins results from a general lowering of vascular disease
or is specific to Alzheimer's disease (maybe by modifying amyloid, the protein that is found in plaques) is unknown. However,
some evidence indicates that maintaining aggressive control of
cholesterol may be an important component in efforts to ward
off unwanted vascular disease and possibly in altering the course
of dementia.

Hypertension and Diabetes

Hypertension and diabetes are other conditions over which you have some control with both medications and lifestyle choices. These are diseases that affect cardiovascular and cerebrovascular function, and these diseases also have an impact on memory function and the possible course of Alzheimer's disease and vascular dementia.

Hypertension is associated with increased risk for stroke and heart attacks. Upwards of 60 percent of people over 65 have hypertension. Furthermore, chronic hypertension during the 40s and 50s is a risk factor for memory decline in later life, and many patients with Alzheimer's disease also have cerebrovascular disease. The evidence is mixed regarding a direct link between hypertension and Alzheimer's disease. A recent Finnish study suggested an association of high systolic blood pressure (but not diastolic blood pressure) and the development of Alzheimer's disease. However, another recent study demonstrated that hypertension in the elderly was not associated with Alzheimer's disease but rather was associated with vascular dementia. In any case, it is clear that control of hypertension is another important factor that can help you manage your memory and mental functions in the long run. Hypertension can be managed through medications as well as through exercise and not smoking.

Diabetes is yet another factor that contributes to loss of memory and mental functioning. Small increases in blood sugar as well as the timing of meals have been shown to improve learning and memory. However, chronic high levels of blood sugar have been associated with lower memory and intellectual function. Diabetics have increased risk for developing memory loss as well as Alzheimer's disease and vascular dementia. This is another factor that you can manage through lifestyle. Eating a healthy diet and exercising clearly help to lower the risk of developing type 2 diabetes. It is important to have regular evaluations for diabetes, especially if you have a family history of the disease, and to treat high blood sugars and diabetes aggressively to further protect your memory and other mental functions.

Anti-Inflammatory Agents

Anti-inflammatory agents may also play a role in protection against Alzheimer's disease but may not help after the disease is clearly established. A large study by the National Institute of Aging between 1955 and 1994 demonstrated that people who regularly used nonsteroidal anti-inflammatory drugs (NSAIDs) (such as ibuprofen, naproxen sodium, and indomethacin) had a lower risk of developing Alzheimer's disease during the course of the study than did persons taking nothing or persons taking acetaminophen. However, trials of prednisone (a steroidal anti-inflammatory agent), naproxen, and refecoxib did not improve memory or functional ability in patients who already had Alzheimer's disease. Current trials are under way to determine if anti-inflammatory agents change the course of Mild Cognitive Impairment. But long-term use of NSAIDs is not recommended as a routine practice. These medications have side effects such as stomach irritation, ulcers, and possible kidney problems that make them poorly tolerated in some and potentially dangerous.

Hormones

Finally, there are many studies on the effects of gonadal hormones, especially replacement therapy in women, on the risk of developing Alzheimer's disease as well as the effect of replacement in those who already have Alzheimer's disease. Several epidemiologic studies suggested that hormone replacement therapy in postmenopausal women reduced the risk of Alzheimer's disease in women, even if the replacement therapy was continued for as short as a period as one year. Estrogen has drawn interest in that it has been shown to promote neuronal sprouting, enhance cholinergic activity in the brain, have anti-inflammatory and anti-oxidative properties, increase cerebral blood flow and glucose metabolism, and lower apolipoprotein levels. However, treatment with estrogen after Alzheimer's disease developed was not helpful. Furthermore, the form of estrogen (e.g., estradiol or conjugated estrogen), the method of delivery (patch or pill), and the relative benefits of combined versus unopposed hormone replacement remain unresolved.

The picture is very unclear and, as with use of anti-inflammatory agents, the risks of long-term use of hormone replacement therapy in women may outweigh the benefits. Indeed, the Women's Health Initiative study of 16,608 women on combined estrogen and progesterone replacement was terminated three years early because the treatment was found to increase the risk of breast cancer, heart disease, and stroke. Furthermore, a report in the *Journal of the American Medical Association* that was published in 2003 suggested that combined hormone replacement (estrogen and progestin) in women 65 and older doubled the risk of developing dementia. It may be that the findings from the earlier studies are a result of the fact that most participants in those studies tended to be better educated and to take better care of themselves. These factors may have accounted for the slowed development of dementia rather than the use of hormone replacement. The final picture is not yet clear.

Hormone replacement therapy in men is also controversial. Starting in their 40s, men have a progressive decline in testosterone in the blood stream. This has led some to propose a condition known as andropause, which is caused by testosterone deficiency. The symptoms of andropause include decreased libido, lack of energy, height loss, irritability, sadness, and decreased strength. However, there are few studies of the effects of androgens on the brain. Some have speculated that androgens may be neuroprotective in men and may explain the lessened prevalence of Alzheimer's disease in men when compared with women before the age of 84 (after which the incidence is the same).

The message from this chapter is simple. Eat well (include fruits, vegetables, and fish in your regular diet and minimize animal fats), exercise, don't smoke (smoking may be associated with mental decline in those who smoke more than 20 cigarettes per day between the ages of 43 and 53), and have regular physicals to monitor blood pressure and blood sugars. This is the same advice that my grandmother gave me as I was growing up.

CHAPTER THIRTEEN

Managing Emotions

We have discussed in detail the mental changes that unfold with normal aging and with disorders of memory. However, thinking and remembering also have emotional components. For example, if I think back to my first and only traffic accident, I cannot only recall a mental image of the accident and its location, but I can also recall the emotions at the time and subsequent anxiety when I drove near the intersection where the accident occurred. Alternatively, when I think back to the first time I saw my wife, Pamela, I can recall the details of where she was in the room and how she was dressed as well as the emotions of attraction that enveloped me as I first laid eyes on her. And there are countless emotions that I experience with no particular referent, such as waking up in a good mood, having a blue day, or worrying when there is no logical basis for worry.

We have not only knowledge and memories of facts, places, times, and people, but we also have memories of emotions. We have positive as well as negative emotions, fleeting as well as enduring emotions. We experience memories that bring joy and memories that bring back sorrow or fear (think back to the death of someone who you cared about). We also have emotional reactions as we anticipate our future (excitement in anticipation of our upcoming wedding, worry about the progress of an illness in someone we love). Emotions may also be connected to changes in the brain. For example, individuals who have sustained a head injury or a stroke or who develop Parkinson's disease are at risk of experiencing depression. Depression may also develop as a reaction to having a serious illness such as cancer or Alzheimer's disease. Emotions are quite complicated and interact in complex ways with memory and with brain structures (specifically, the amygdala).

Often we talk of ourselves as being "stressed" by events around us such as our increasing forgetfulness, having too much to do, failing at something that matters to us, or even succeeding. Stress is often used to refer to either an internal physical response (feeling nervous, or feeling pounding or discomfort in the chest) or a psychological response (anticipation, dread, worry, avoidance, escape). Stresses may be nonspecific, or they may induce specific emotions such as anxiety or depression. Many who have memory loss experience symptoms of anxiety or depression as do those who care for them. Therefore, this chapter will focus on describing depression, anxiety, and stress, and on ways to manage these emotions.

Depression

Depression is generally believed to be the most common emotional challenge of elderly people without memory loss. Self-rating scales suggest that 15 to 20 percent of those over 65 and living independently experience depressive symptoms. We know that about six million people in the United States suffer from depression. But these statistics may be only the tip of the iceberg. A recent study suggested that as many as 50 percent of patients in primary care practices who had depressive symptoms were not diagnosed.

Depression is associated with increased life stress and daily hassles. For example, depression may develop as a result of a loved one dying, the loss of a job, divorce, being injured in an accident, or being diagnosed with a neurological disease such as Alzheimer's disease. We may become depressed at the loss or anticipated loss of an ability and of self-determination. Caregivers may experience depression as a result of lack of companionship, affectional deprivation, or having to take on things they never did in the past, such as managing finances or a checkbook, doing laundry, maintaining a care schedule, or preparing meals.

Depression is also associated with decreased frequency of social contacts, poor self-esteem, decreased comfort in interpersonal events, and diminished enjoyment of pleasant activities. Additionally, there is a clear association between pain or physical illness and depression, with increased severity of pain and illness contributing to increased severity of depression. Medical conditions such as Alzheimer's disease, Parkinson's disease, hypothyroidism, Cushing's disease, stroke, and cardiovascular disease also contribute to depression. As discussed in chapter 12, depression appears to be a risk factor for developing Alzheimer's disease. Despite amazing resilience following loss, as many as 25 percent of elders experience clinical depression during the first year of bereavement after the death of a loved one. Depression is clearly a pervasive and often unrecognized complication of living and dealing with life's experiences.

SYMPTOMS OF DEPRESSION

It is no wonder that depression has been referred to as the "common cold" of mental health. Symptoms of depression vary across individuals but often include changes in emotion (sadness, guilt, anxiety), behavior (withdrawal from others, tearfulness), physiology (fatigue, changes in sleep and/or appetite), and thought patterns (loss of pleasure, feelings of worthlessness, hopelessness). There are also many gradations in severity of depression from mild demoralization to severe withdrawal from the world (spending large periods of time not

TABLE 7

Circle all items that pertain to you and have been present for at least two weeks

1. Withdrawal from friends and family

2. Withdrawal from usual activities

3. Tire easily

4. Excessive sleep

5. Too little sleep

6. Premature awakening

7. Poor concentration

8. Self-destructive thoughts

9. Tearful

10. Marked lack of pleasure in life

11. Sadness

12. Depressed mood nearly every day

13. Restlessness

14. Feeling slowed down

15. Feeling worthless

getting dressed and not going out of the house) and constant desire for death. Interestingly, many people with depression do not feel depressed or sad and may even be surprised if told they are depressed. Depression is a state of sadness that does not pass in a matter of hours or a couple of days. It is more than being "blue." Depression is a change in mood that endures for at least a matter of weeks and can last for months or even years.

Table 7 lists a number of symptoms that are associated with depression. You can use the table as a self-test to determine whether you have symptoms that are consistent with depression. If you circle "marked loss of pleasure in life," "self-destructive thoughts," or "sadness," or you circle at least five items, you may be depressed. If you feel that you may be depressed, it is important to seek counsel from a professional whom you trust.

TREATMENT FOR DEPRESSION

There are two main strategies for treating depression: medications and counseling. Both can be effective in managing depression, as can a combination of the two. Common medications for treating depression include Prozac, Zoloft, Celexa, Lexipro, Effexor, Remeron, Wellbutrin, and Desyrel, to name a few. The choice of the correct medication needs to be determined by a physician or a psychiatrist. However, management of a depression demands more than use of medications. Indeed, many depressions respond very well to non-medical treatments such as counseling or support groups. Furthermore, medications are often most effective when accompanied by counseling. Depression presents another example of a circumstance that we may have to deal with through our own actions. Although there are medications that can help, we still have to manage thoughts and lifestyle because medications do not cure depression without our participation.

The fundamental psychological treatment for depression consists of trying to reestablish a sense of life and direction.

Therapies often focus on reducing self-defeating thoughts, such as "I am worthless," and behaviors, such as withdrawal from friends by refusing invitations, that feed the depression. I often call the treatment for depression "Listerine Therapy" in that it may taste bad, but it is good for you. Treatment is directed at helping you to overcome the inertia of the withdrawal and inactivity that accompanies depression. The first step in managing depression is to become active and get moving again in a physical and social world. Depression makes you lose track of joy and interests. Treating depression requires that you return to your past interests and pleasures even if you don't want to.

One of the skills that I hope you have developed from reading this book is that of a good calendar habit. A good calendar can help treat depression because life fills in around what is in our calendar. If you are blue or depressed, start putting events in your calendar (lunch with friends, shopping, reading a good book) that were sources of interest and active involvement for you when you were not depressed. Over time, increase the number of these pleasing activities, and use your calendar as a personal contract with yourself to engage in activities. The essence of this plan is not doing what you want to do but rather doing what you have planned to do and used to enjoy. You do not have to have a good memory to follow this plan; you only need a good calendar habit.

Anxiety

If depression is the most common emotional challenge we all face, anxiety runs a close second. Anxiety, like depression, affects your whole being and has physiological, behavioral, and psychological components. If you have ever been afraid, recall both how you felt and how your body reacted and you will know the "symptoms" of anxiety. Anxiety induces a mental and physiological state that is similar to fear. However, anxiety often does not have a specific, concrete, external object as does fear. (I am afraid of the snake in the living room, but I am anxious about a snake that I might encounter in my backyard.). There are no life-or-death implications of the snake we never encounter or of having to give a speech, but we can become anxious if we anticipate something bad or dangerous or if we have to talk in front of others. Anxiety is produced by a symbolic, vague, distant, anticipated, or unrecognized danger. We feel anxious about "losing control" or have the feeling that "something bad will happen."

SYMPTOMS OF ANXIETY

Anxiety is often associated with depression, and the two may coexist and be difficult to differentiate. Anxiety also appears to increase with stress and daily hassles. The symptoms of anxiety are complex. Anxiety produces physical changes such as rapid heartbeat, muscle tension, dry mouth, queasy stomach, and/or sweating. Anxiety also produces behavioral symptoms such as avoidance, reduction in the efficiency of thought, and inhibition of expression, all of which are maladaptive. Psychologically, anxiety is perceived as a feeling of apprehension and uneasiness. In its most extreme presentation, anxiety can produce a feeling of extreme detachment or fear of dying or going crazy.

Anxiety may range in severity from a twinge of uneasiness to a panic attack. Panic attacks may be experienced as heart palpitations, disorientation, and terror. They are often "out of the blue" and may cause fear that one is having a heart attack as the symptoms can be very similar. Anxiety may be spontaneous or anticipatory. Symptoms may last from a few minutes to hours. Anxiety may display itself as worry or dread. Anxiety is likely to arise from small hassles (not being able to find the TV remote) as well as from major stressors (losing one's job, death of a loved one). Anxiety often serves as a signal of anticipated, imagined, or real danger. It is our internal danger signal system that helps us escape or avoid dangerous objects or situations and keeps us out of harm's way. Unfortunately, this signal can work too well and induce us to avoid or escape situations that are not dangerous. For example, anxiety might keep you from asking out a person you're interested in or interviewing for a job you really want.

Although some anxiety is appropriate and reasonable in certain situations, it sometimes becomes extreme and may interfere with significant aspects of our life. Extreme or clinically significant anxiety is marked by its intensity and duration. It often leads to avoidance and/or escape. For example, someone who is anxious about a medical test such as having blood drawn to determine if he or she has cancer may wait too long to have the test and thereby undermine treatments that might have helped earlier. Or a person may fear changes in memory and thus wait too long to seek adequate assessment, thereby reducing the control he or she has over current and future memory loss.

FORMS THAT ANXIETY MAY TAKE

There are various disorders of anxiety recognized by mental health professionals. Table 8 provides a summary and brief description of the major forms in which anxiety may present. Most of us have some of these characteristics at one time or another, but the duration and intensity of the emotion can make anxiety disruptive.

TREATMENTS FOR ANXIETY

Treating anxiety is easy, in principle. Anxiety can be decreased by reducing physiological reactivity (that is, by managing and/or reducing the symptoms). This may be accomplished through induced relaxation with techniques such as massage, hypnosis, or deep breathing, or by means of medications such as antidepressant medications (Paxil, Effexor) or

TABLE 8

FORMS OF ANXIETY

Panic Disorder
— intense overwhelming fear often without obvious cause

Agoraphobia
— fear of open spaces which often leads one to be homebound

Social Phobia
— possibly a form of shyness

Specific Phobia
— snakes, closed spaces, dentists, heights

Generalized Anxiety
— persistent and maladaptive worry

Obsessive-Compulsive Disorder
— spending many hours cleaning, checking the locks

Post-traumatic Stress Disorder
— reaction to a severe trauma (surviving a hurricane, assault, rape)

Acute Stress Disorder
— similar to Post-traumatic Stress Disorder but resolves in four weeks

Anxiety, Disorder due to a
General Medical Condition
— hyperthyroidism, pulmonary disease

Substance-Induced Anxiety Disorder
— overdose of caffeine or other substance

anxiety-reducing medications (BuSpar, Xanax, Ativan, Valium). Anxiety may also be managed by gradually preventing avoidance or escape while you are in the presence of the anxiety-arousing situation. This is referred to as "desensitization." For example, if individuals were fearful of dogs, they would engage in gradual or intense exposure to dogs (preferably ones that are safe) until they were comfortable with a variety of dogs. Finally, anxiety may be managed by altering what we say to ourselves or how we think about events and situations that make us anxious. For example, when confronted by a difficult situation (such as going on a job interview or giving a speech), we can encourage ourselves or "psyche ourselves up." If we spill our coffee first thing in the morning, we can remind ourselves that the entire day is not ruined. We do not have to be liked by everyone, and we don't have to perform each task we undertake with perfection.

In short, the techniques used to treat anxiety include relaxation, physical exercise, imagery, desensitization, challenging mistaken beliefs, assertion training, and/or medications. Fortunately, we can usually manage anxiety and depression by participating in enjoyable activities that may help manage symptoms directly (desensitization, relaxation, or exercise) or in activities that are so involving that they distract us from anxiety-provoking thoughts and block rumination. Table 9 presents examples of some useful activities to consider. This list is not exhaustive.

Stress

People who are depressed or anxious often refer to themselves as being "stressed." Although some stress is probably good for us, constant stress can be debilitating and can be the precipitant for developing depression and/or anxiety. There are three important factors to consider when trying to understand stress.

TABLE 9

SUGGESTIONS OF POSSIBLE PLEASURABLE ACTIVITIES

- ☐ Exercise
- ☐ Watch sports in person
- ☐ Watch sports on TV
- ☐ Go on a long walk
- ☐ Walk on the beach
- ☐ Take a dance class
- ☐ Take an exercise class
- ☐ Ride a bicycle
- ☐ Ride a stationary cycle
- ☐ Walk on a treadmill
- ☐ Walk at a mall
- ☐ Do a swamp tour
- ☐ Go canoeing
- ☐ Go kayaking
- ☐ Garden
- ☐ Clean

- ☐ Shop
- ☐ Buy flowers for yourself
- ☐ Spend less time alone
- ☐ Visit your children
- ☐ Take a day trip
- ☐ Take a cruise
- ☐ Take a vacation
- ☐ Volunteer to help others
- ☐ Relax in a natural setting

- ☐ Do yoga
- ☐ Meditate
- ☐ Pray
- ☐ Go to church
- ☐ Do relaxation exercises
- ☐ Spend time outside
- ☐ Laugh

- ☐ Read
- ☐ Listen to a book on tape
- ☐ Listen to music
- ☐ Play a musical instrument
- ☐ Watch videos

- ☐ Take a class
- ☐ Write letters
- ☐ Write poetry
- ☐ Write in a journal
- ☐ Draw
- ☐ Paint
- ☐ Work with wood
- ☐ Do ceramics
- ☐ Do crafts
- ☐ Do needlework

- ☐ Get a pet
- ☐ Spend time with your pet
- ☐ Get an aquarium

First, stress is a response to threatening or fearful events that may be either real (the lion in the bedroom) or imagined/anticipated (having symptoms that may be signs of serious illness). Second, stress is adaptive and serves our innate need for survival. By anticipating danger we can either escape or avoid a dangerous object or situation. Stress is the activation of our danger signal system. Third, stress fuels our "fight-or-flight" response. That is, stress activates our body to either stand and fight or flee danger.

COPING WITH STRESS

The objective in coping with stress is to manage rather than to eliminate stress. You cannot eliminate stress from your life. Stress is a normal reaction to both positive and negative life experiences, such as graduating from school, raising children, death of a spouse, or retirement. Stress is not a global response but rather a set of behaviors, thoughts, and reactions. If we break stress down into components, we can better develop strategies for managing stressful situations. We need to begin by focusing our awareness on the first, low intensity cues that let us know we are feeling stressed and implement plans and strategies to manage the stress early in the process. If we wait for the heat of battle before trying to cope, we will be much less successful. For example, if I have to give a talk on Friday afternoon, it is too late to start preparing on Friday morning. Indeed, the main message of this book has been to start planning and managing early. Memory loss is a major stressor for those who experience the loss and also for the people who live with or care about them. That's why we don't want to wait for memory loss to be debilitating before starting to cope with it. Seek assessment early. Plan ahead. Consider the needs of both the person with the memory loss and the potential caregiver(s) in the plan.

PROBLEM-FOCUSED STRESS MANAGEMENT

There are two general styles of coping with stress, and both are important. First, there is what is called the problem-focused or instrumental style of coping. This method involves gathering and using information. It involves planning and the use of logic and reasoning to manage stressful situations. The specific steps for problem-focused coping include:

1. Gathering information
2. Problem-solving
3. Communication
4. Time management
5. Taking direct action.

Reading this book and applying what works for you is an example of problem-focused coping. If you have memory loss, studying memory and learning all you can about memory loss will help you cope with the stress. If you have cancer, learning

TABLE 10

STEPS IN PROBLEM SOLVING

— What is my concern?

— What do I want?

— What can I do?

— What might happen?

— What is my decision?

— Do it!

— Did it work?

— What changes, if any, do I need to make?

all you can about cancer will help you manage the stress. Decide on goals you want to reach, and break them into small, manageable steps. Then start moving forward one step at a time. The steps you might wish to consider in solving a difficult problem are listed as questions to ask yourself in Table 10. Pick something easy and accomplishable (exercise for 20 minutes three times a week) to help build your confidence before you tackle harder problems. Refine your plan as needed.

EMOTION-FOCUSED STRESS MANAGEMENT

Emotion-focused stress management requires using strategies to manage your emotions rather than gathering information. Emotion-focused strategies include questioning meaning ("Why is this happening to me?"). Support groups often assist with managing emotions in that they allow social comparisons ("I am not alone"). For example, I have long been involved with a support group for couples in which the husband, wife, or parent has mild memory loss (either Mild Cognitive Impairment or early Alzheimer's disease). These groups are very effective for gaining information about diseases of memory, but more importantly, they provide support and reduce the isolation for both the person with memory loss and the caregiver. These groups also help the participants to accept their lot (another emotion-focused strategy) without giving up. These groups also help couples learn how to compromise (another emotion-focused strategy) rather than fight about issues.

The group members have engaged in activities such as going to lunch or going to a movie (diverting attention away from the problem for a time). Some members have engaged in denial (deny that memory changes are indications of Alzheimer's disease). As long as the persons are actively doing what they need to do (such as being in the group, managing lifestyle, and taking appropriate medications), they reduce their stress and the denial can be helpful. Some of the

TABLE 11

STEPS TO COPE WITH STRESS

Preparing for the stressor
- — What do I have to do?
- — Develop a plan
- — Avoid negative self-statements and self-criticism
- — Minimize worry

Confronting and handling the stressor
- — Psych yourself up
- — Take one step at a time
- — Stay relevant
- — Focus on the task at hand
- — Tenseness is a cue for the need to cope
- — Reduce tenseness by relaxing – e.g., take a deep breath

Coping with being overwhelmed
- — When fear comes, pause
- — Focus on the present
- — Focus on what you have to do
- — Expect tension and fear
- — Manage the fear and tension

Reinforcing yourself
- — I did it!
- — It wasn't as bad as I expected
- — Be pleased with yourself
- — Tell others about your success
- — Do something good to yourself

group members have gone somewhere alone to scream and let out their frustration. Finally, members have engaged in many forms of relaxation (massage, deep breathing exercises, using relaxation tapes and videos) to induce periods of calm so the stress is not constant. All of these strategies are examples of ways to reduce stress by focusing on reducing the intensity of emotions.

Table 11 presents a guide for managing stress. The elements in the table engage both problem- and emotion-focused coping strategies for managing stress. Donald Michenbaum has labeled this process as being "stress inoculation training."

CHAPTER FOURTEEN

Managing Your Future Today

In its earliest stages, Alzheimer's disease is relatively benign and mostly causes inconvenience
and annoyance. As the disease progresses, it causes
increasing adaptive and mental impairment until
near its middle stage when it causes substantial disability. Alzheimer's disease becomes more prevalent
with age. For people who live into their 60s, the
prevalence is less than 5 percent. However, for those
who live to be 85 to 90, the prevalence increases to nearly
50 percent, and by 95, the prevalence increases to about 60
percent.

Forgetfulness is usually the earliest sign of the disease
(although different presentations such as greater language
impairment than memory impairment are not uncommon). In
the beginning one usually becomes less able to manage higher
level finances such as preparing taxes, balancing a checkbook, or
paying bills. Further into the disease, managing home life
becomes increasingly difficult. For example, keeping things
organized, shopping, preparing meals, traveling independently,
and driving become more and more difficult and finally fail. As

the disease progresses, receiving care, monitoring, and supervision becomes increasingly necessary. In middle stages of the disease, self-care becomes an increasing challenge, so more and more external assistance may be needed. In short, the disease unfolds over a trajectory of years to decades. Fortunately, the progression is typically slow, even without the use of medications. If you act early, time is your ally because you can plan your own future. If you wait too long, others must do the planning for you.

Most of us have a long-range financial plan to cover financial needs after retirement. We buy insurance in case we are confronted by fire, floods, hurricanes, or death. We plan ahead for our funerals. It seems to me that we should also put together a plan that will act as a "safety net" in case we become cognitively or adaptively impaired with neurological or medical diseases that rob us of skills or mobility. It is far better to plan ahead than to have to react to an unanticipated outcome or crisis. Planning allows control and self-determination. A plan for possible changes in mental and physical abilities can be made at any time during our life and revised as necessary for changing circumstances. Although many are planning ahead these days by buying long-term care insurance, this does not help with difficult and emotional decisions that may have to be made such as when to stop driving or whether to move to an assisted living facility. It is never too early to begin to outline such a plan. There are so many who still do not have a living will despite strong feelings that they do not want to be on artificial life support in a vegetative state. It's a good idea to make a living will a part of this plan, just in case.

It is imperative to work out a safety net if you develop Mild Cognitive Impairment or you have a strong family history of memory loss. Your plans should be determined while memory loss is mild and judgment and reasoning are strong. Decide how you would like to spend your time and where and by whom care

TABLE 12

ISSUES TO CONSIDER IN LONG-TERM PLANNING

Who will decide?
— Durable Power of Attorney
— Trusts
— Guardianships

Living wills

Do not resuscitate (DNR) orders

Driving

Cooking

Handling finances

Having a credit card

Doing the checkbook

Assisted Living

will be provided if you cannot care for yourself. Specify your specific desires about handling serious or terminal illnesses, such as whether you want mechanical life supports and whether you want to be resuscitated should your heart stop beating or your breathing stop. Decide under what circumstances you should stop driving, stop doing the checkbook, begin to use companions, or make a move into an assisted living facility or skilled nursing home.

It is vital that your plans for your future and care options be in writing. As a written document, it will serve as a permanent external memory aid so you can remind yourself of the decisions you have made and the ways you want the decisions to be carried out should your memory fail. This document should be periodically reviewed because the details will probably change as you age or face illnesses such as Mild Cognitive Impairment, Alzheimer's disease, or cancer. It is important that those closest to you have access to this document as well so that they can know and carry out your wishes if your memory begins to fail. Table 12 presents an outline of the elements that should be considered in a plan that determines how you want your life managed in serious illness or if you ever become demented.

Voluntary Transfer of Decision Making

DURABLE POWERS OF ATTORNEY

Who will make decisions for you if you are unable to? Don't take it for granted that the person you want to manage your life will be able to. A durable power of attorney is a legal document specifying the circumstances for voluntary transfer of decision making and to whom the assignment is to be made. Durable powers of attorney allow the voluntary transfer of decision making in the event that you become incapacitated by events such as strokes, heart attacks, or dementia and cannot make decisions for yourself. These documents should provide for a selected representative, often a spouse or children, to manage financial matters as well as healthcare decisions. A durable power of attorney appoints someone to act as your "attorney in fact" to make medical and/or financial decisions in your place. This document is different from a power of attorney which allows for a time-limited representation for specific decisions, such as if I would give my wife my power of attorney to sell our house.

TRUSTS

Trusts or living trusts are more complex legal documents and are often set up during estate planning. Trusts may be either revocable or irrevocable. The latter is ordinarily a device for the very rich to minimize tax liability. A revocable trust appoints someone as a trustee to manage your assets and property. However, there is a clause in this document allowing the trustor (the one who initiates the document) the right to revoke the trust at any time. An irrevocable trust does not contain this clause. Trusts and durable powers of attorney are complex legal documents and should be worked out in collaboration with an attorney.

The advantage of a durable power of attorney or trust is that it provides a mechanism allowing a person you choose to act on your behalf if you become incapacitated. These documents generally avoid the need for court interventions such as guardianships (discussed next). A durable power of attorney or a trust requires advanced planning because it has to be enacted while one has the memory and mental and legal capacity to make his or her own decisions. They are best completed before one develops diagnosable Alzheimer's disease or another dementing condition. They require consultation with an attorney, and if they are to cover changes that may occur in aging, it is preferable to use an attorney who is familiar with elder law and related issues in the state in which you reside. Clearly, having a predetermined transfer of powers is advantageous psychologically, economically, and practically. As is the case with buying insurance, durable powers of attorneys are documents for peace of mind that we hope we will never have to use.

Involuntary Transfers of Decision Making through Guardianships

Guardianships are actions involving the court and are required when a person is already incapacitated (with dementia, coma, or delirium). Court proceedings to establish a guardianship are enacted as "protective." A guardian is a person who is appointed by a court to manage all or part of an incapacitated person's affairs after a court-ordered evaluation and formal hearing before a judge. A guardian is appointed when a person does not have sufficient mental capacity (due to conditions such as mental illness, mental retardation, or Alzheimer's disease) to understand and make informed decisions such as forming contracts, deciding where to live, or deciding on appropriate treatment for an illness or disease.

Guardianships are necessary when a person loses capacity to make decisions and has not planned ahead by prior establishment of durable powers of attorney or a trust while legally competent. A guardianship is formed when a court appoints a surrogate decision maker who is given the legal right and responsibility to make decisions about where the incapacitated person can live, how to dispense money and manage property, what medical decisions need to be made, and so forth. These legal proceedings are usually conducted before a probate court of the county in which the person lives. This process is expensive and may cost several thousand dollars. Furthermore, being involved in court proceedings can be very stressful and, in the case of those with illnesses such as Alzheimer's disease, occurs when the person cannot understand why this is happening to them and may think they are being taken advantage of or in legal trouble. Therefore, it is much better to establish durable powers of attorney as "insurance" in order to try to avoid this emotionally and financially difficult outcome should you become incapacitated.

The Living Will

Most states have enacted laws to allow the "right-to-die." These laws were motivated by the famous case of Karen Ann Quinlan in 1976. Right-to-die laws allow you or your empowered representative to shut off life support machines should your condition become hopeless, if that is your wish. A living will is the mechanism to convey your wish not to continue to live if you have a terminal illness and can only be kept alive with life support machines or are in a vegetative medical state. You will be kept comfortable and pain free until your death. A living will makes your wishes known to your family and physician and is a legal document that is drawn up in consultation with an attorney. A physician who complies with this directive cannot be sued for honoring those wishes. This document should be a part of your medical file and discussed with your primary care physician as well as your attorney before there is a need for it as part of the safety net you build for your own future.

Do Not Resuscitate Orders

You may also wish to consider a do-not-resuscitate (DNR) order. This is often confused with a living will but does not cover the same issues. A DNR provides medical workers with a clear directive about whether or not you wish to be revived if you stop breathing. In effect, it directs emergency service personnel not to administer cardiopulmonary resuscitation (CPR) or electrical stimulation to restart your breathing or your heart if it were to stop on its own. Obviously, this is a document that needs to be carefully considered and is typically formed by persons with serious and often terminal illnesses or progressive neurological disorders. The decision to enact a DNR may change with age or disease states. I have had clients in their late 80s and 90s who are fearful of death and do not have a DNR order. On the other hand, another client in her early 90s had her DRN laminated and wears it on a chain under her blouse.

Decision Making about Daily Activities

It is interesting that people commonly make detailed funeral plans, but we fail to make plans to cover everyday life situations such as how to decide when it is time to stop driving or what circumstances under which we and our family would be better served by using companions or moving into facilities with assisted living or skilled nursing care. Despite the lack of formal or legal processes to protect our rights and allow us to plan our own course in terms of our everyday activities, such as driving, in the event of mental or physical decline, we still have avenues through which we can manage to do prudent planning for ourselves in these areas.

Creating the right safety net for someone vulnerable to progressive mental decline should involve the consideration of many issues. These issues are important to discuss with your spouse and family or close friends. The discussions can be difficult, but the result is that you can gain control in advance of how difficult situations may be handled based on your wishes. The details of how you want certain situations handled are best put in writing for future reference should they be needed. Discussing these issues early in the course of possible mental decline, such as Mild Cognitive Impairment, and making a plan can provide you with control and save your family agonizing decisions at times of great stress.

Driving

We all want to drive as long as we are safe drivers. And we would all probably agree that we should stop driving if we no longer have the skills behind the wheel of a car (or golf cart or motorized scooter) that allow us to be safe. But progressive or sudden changes in mental and motor functions increase the risk of driving. How can you decide when it is time to stop driving? I often hear clients say, "I will know when it is time." However, the essential dilemma presented by dementing conditions is that, despite good intentions, you probably will *not* know when it is time to make the decision to stop driving. Poor insight into one's deficiencies is a cardinal sign of most dementias, as well as is poor judgment. Furthermore, short-term memory loss means you may not remember your close calls, your accidents (such as the client mentioned earlier who had five accidents in the previous month but could not recall any of them and thought she was a safe driver), or a large number of persons who honk at you because of poor decision making in the car. Therefore, a decision needs to be made early about how to decide when to stop driving (well before the actual decision of stopping driving) and put in writing.

Consider the following suggestions as guidelines for deciding that you are no longer safe to drive:

1. If you get lost in the car while driving in familiar locations, you should stop driving.
2. If a trusted friend or relative is afraid to ride with you, it is time to stop driving.
3. If you confuse the brake and the gas pedal, you should stop driving.
4. If you confuse the symbols on the gear shift (reverse and drive), you should stop driving.
5. If you make bad judgments behind the wheel (do not use a turn signal consistently or leave it blinking when you are not turning, turn into oncoming traffic, drive at inappropriate speeds, keep hitting the curb while driving), you should stop driving.
6. If you constantly have others honking their horns at you, you should stop driving.
7. Consider having a formal driving evaluation by a certified evaluator if you have any changes in memory or mental skills to help with this decision. If you fail this test, you should stop driving.

Include in your written plan the incidents that are critical errors (driving too fast, turning into oncoming traffic) that you know would make a driver unsafe. Work out this agreement with someone you trust and put the agreement with your important papers. You may also wish to appoint some agreed upon person to tell you that you should stop driving because you are no longer safe by your own prior agreement. This decision may be enacted either with the assistance of a relative or of a professional who knows of the agreement. Finally, decide on how you will manage if you can no longer drive. Make tentative plans for alternative forms of transportation so you do not become homebound.

Other Areas of Potential Difficulty

When should you stop using the stove and /or the microwave? You may forget that something is on the stove and start a fire. You may put materials in a microwave or an oven that will start a fire. When should you no longer have credit cards? I have known of people who have given $30 tips for a $10 meal. I have seen people who were previously extremely responsible with their money run up thousands of dollars in credit card debts. When should you give up preparing the taxes? When should you stop doing a checkbook? When should you no longer be able to access your main financial accounts? When should someone else manage your medications? When should you stop traveling?

All of these difficult decisions may need to be made at some point if you develop a dementia. The decisions are not always clear-cut. They may involve sequential steps based on your retained abilities. However, the process of making these decisions goes much smoother for those who have thought these issues through and have developed a general plan and committed it to writing.

You will need not only to monitor yourself in these areas but to have someone you trust monitor you also in case you are unable to either perceive or remember your own limitations. Monitor how well you do a checkbook, safely prepare food, and reliably take your medications. If you make mistakes, develop a plan that will eliminate the mistakes (use a timer, hire a companion, move to assisted living). Also, consider having someone else who you trust do high finances and manage your checkbook if you are struggling. Reduce the credit limits on your credit cards to the amount of money you can afford to lose, or destroy all credit cards and cancel the accounts. Carry only as much cash with you in your purse or wallet as you can afford to lose. Keep important papers safely secure and where someone trusted can always get at them (such as in a safety deposit box to which your spouse or trusted companion has a key or knows the location of the key).

Assisted Living

Assisted living can be used to manage daily living for those of us who have a mental or physical impairment that prevents us from independently caring for some particular function for ourselves. For example, not being able to manage a checkbook means that you need assistance with doing your checkbook. Not being able to drive means that you need someone else to assist you with getting from one place to another that is too far to walk. Sometimes, assistance is provided by a family member such as a spouse or a child. If you have the financial assets or if you have good long-term care insurance, you can hire the help you need. If the assistance is greater than a family member can or will manage, then you need assistance from another source.

Assistance can take many forms. For example, friends may help. Neighbors may help. Compassionate groups and organizations, such as church groups, may help. Alternatively, you may prefer more formal systems for assistance that would require paying someone to help. For example, you might hire a companion or a home health service. Or you may prefer to use day programs that provide not only necessary supervision but also stimulation and rewarding (to you) activities. Some may choose to move to a formal assisted living facility or to a skilled nursing facility, where the available care is extensive. How you decide to obtain the care you need is up to you and those who care about you. Put the tentative plan in writing and review it periodically, hoping that you never have to use it but enjoying the confidence that comes from knowing that you have a clear plan.

Development of a plan for use of assistance often needs to be creative and is best done by pre-planning. As much as some of us feel that we would never want to use any resources outside of family, extracting a promise such as never to use a skilled nursing facility for our care only makes things worse for the caregiver, and possibly the care receiver, should such a need arise. We are always best in a familiar environment with familiar loved ones as caregivers, but this is not always possible. Early discussion of possible ways to manage our care and of the triggers that will start the conditions in the plan for incorporating various levels of assistance can save a great deal of anxiety, anger, and guilt. An example may help clarify this point.

I assessed a 70-year-old single man who had mild Alzheimer's disease. After the assessment we discussed his strengths and weaknesses. He had few local supports, and we discussed his prognosis which was for continued and progressive decline over the course of months to years. He decided to move from his house to a large retirement community as part of his plan to remain as independent as possible for as long as possible. He chose the particular retirement community because it had care ranging from independent living to assisted living to skilled nursing care as continuous services. He moved into an independent apartment and used a home health aid and a companion to help him with meal preparation and shopping. His son, who lived in another state, managed his finances. We also discussed his interests and needs. He was physically very active and wanted to keep being able to play tennis, play billiards, and ride his bicycle. He had the financial resources to hire a companion who played tennis and billiards with him most days of the week (so he could not forget to play often). In short, we kept his activities intact so that as his memory loss progressed, he continued to do what brought him joy.

As his illness progressed over the next couple of years, he was no longer able to drive, shop, or prepare meals. He expanded companion time in order to keep him in his apartment, continue with his activities, and go on rides and out to lunch. He developed close relationships with his companions. Although he was unable to tell someone what he did each day or each week, he kept his life full of the joyful activities that were meaningful to him because of the companions. He also kept himself out of the assisted living facility for several years because he had set up such good routines and supports earlier in the course of his illness. He did not have to remember what to do to enjoy life.

I have worked with several other individuals and couples to make creative use of companions and routines to keep their life intact and to delay the need to move into more structured care. These plans need to be flexible and structured in light of the background, needs, joys, activities, and desires of both the person who has memory loss and his or her primary caregivers. The plan needs to be fluid and flexible, and it should be periodically revised. It is important to remember that if you wait until you need the elements of the plan, you may be too impaired to institute and develop a plan to secure your own future.

CHAPTER FIFTEEN

Final Comments on Putting It All Together

We have covered a lot of territory. As I reflect on what I have written, the essential question that I am left with is this: Can we age "successfully" as our memory becomes less efficient as a consequence of aging or under the more trying circumstances of developing a memory disorder? I hope I have convinced you that you can definitely manage memory changes successfully by planning well ahead. Practicing good memory hygiene will help you create a good safety net that addresses your personal joys, skills, and needs. If you have any concerns, seek the counsel of a memory expert as early as possible.

I also hope I have convinced you that you need to do all of this *before* you need it. Let's review the main principles that will allow you to develop a plan suitable for managing your own future.

Memory Is Complex

Memory consists of a myriad of abilities. This is fortunate because even those with clinically significant memory loss often retain many kinds of memory that they can still use. The main challenge is managing short-term memory. This means managing new learning. We need to make use of other memory systems and other mental skills to cleverly compensate for challenges in new learning as we age or if we develop a memory disorder.

Although Aging Does Not Destine Loss of Memory, the Efficiency of Memory Declines as a Natural Consequence of Aging

I do not have the same efficiency of memory now as I did 10 years ago. I will have a less efficient memory in 10 more years. This means I will have to spend more of my time and energy organizing my life and using supports for my memory as I grow older. There are no shortcuts. Still, this doesn't mean that I will develop memory loss or Alzheimer's disease. Indeed, if I live to be 90, I will have about a 50 percent chance of having a normal memory—for a 90-year-old.

There Are Many Things That Increase the Likelihood of Forgetting

Forgetting is a natural component of memory. However, we can manage many elements in our life that will help us to reduce the amount of forgetting that we will do. For example, we can keep our living and work spaces more organized. We can reduce clutter. We can help increase our attention by minimizing distractions. We can also give our attention a boost by doing more demanding mental tasks when we are more efficient, which is in the mornings for many but later in the day for others. We can manage our use of drugs and alcohol since they reduce the efficiency of memory and attention. And we can keep our vision and hearing as sharp as possible with corrective eyewear and hearing aids, if necessary.

Anticipate and Plan for Likely Areas Where Memory May Be Unreliable

Our short-term memory becomes less efficient in a number of areas as we age. We may sometimes forget what people tell us. We may forget appointments if we don't write them down and then refer to our calendar to remind us. We may have increasing difficulty following complex sets of characters and plots in novels and movies. We may sometimes forget where we parked our car. We may forget phone messages and forget names even more than we used to. We may repeat ourselves to our spouse or friends because we forget that we already told them something. And we may sometimes even forget that we forget.

By using external memory aids, you can help yourself on all of these fronts. Whether you're simply anticipating the memory changes of aging or are experiencing the early stages of a memory disorder, it is best to implement your personal safety net while your memory is normal for your age. As I mentioned early in the book, for nearly all of us, our memory is the best it will ever be right now. You will not be able to develop the skills you'll need to manage your memory if you wait until you need those skills. If you ever grow concerned about your memory, it is important to seek a professional consultation with an expert in memory assessment and treatment as soon as possible. Still, I hope I have convinced you that you needn't fear Mild Cognitive Impairment. This is a phase of memory decline in which you have a great deal of control and can develop the skills you need to create a safety net for the future.

Use Cleverness and Long-Term Memory

It is our short-term memory that is the culprit, making new learning more and more difficult as we age or develop memory loss. Therefore, we need to seek stimulation by doing what we like and know well. We also need to develop routines and set goals that are based on what we want and need to do with our time. It is extremely valuable to create and re-create our life history in a concrete form. To enhance our life history, we can find and organize our life's memorabilia, such as the pictures we all have stuck in boxes in our closets or garage. In these ways and others that are personal to each individual, we can establish multiple cues to trigger our memory over time.

Implement the General Rules for Managing Memory

Memory loss cannot be cured. Therefore, we need to use our remaining skills and external memory aids liberally. Now is the time to develop the skills and habit of implementing memory aids so that we will have them when we really need them. You might start by beginning a calendar in which you write down what is important and also what is pleasurable in your life. You can develop the habit of using a tape recorder. It is important to learn to manage fatigue and stress, and to keep your learning sessions short and frequent. Develop a plan to become and remain more organized. Now is also the time to develop the habit of spending more time and more effort with those things that are important for you to remember.

Use External Memory Aids

Developing a good calendar habit is key to getting organized. It's useful to keep both a master calendar that stays at home and a daily calendar or appointment book that you carry with you at all times. Start using a digital watch and clock. Begin a diary or journal to recall trips, family visits, or other things in your life that are important to you. Use timers and to-do lists. Create a take-away spot where you put everything that needs to leave the house with you, and develop the habit of using that spot without fail. And while you're at it, decide on a place for everything and develop the habit of putting everything in its place—every time. Unfortunately, good intentions do not make for good memory. We cannot always count on our short-term memory, but external memory aids can keep us efficient by using other skills and parts of our memory.

Manage Biology

Current studies indicate that fruits, vegetables, and fish contain substances that may help our mind and memory function more efficiently, so it only makes sense to eat a diet rich in these foods most of the time. We also know that cardiovascular health and blood-sugar levels can affect how successfully our memory ages, so we need to exercise most days of the week—and keep our exercise plan in our daily calendar. It's important to include both cardiovascular and strength training in our exercise routine.

Plan Ahead

I already have insurance. I won't wait for a hurricane before I buy hurricane insurance because I live in Florida. Of course, I never want to collect on my hurricane insurance, but I'm ready just in case. I have also been planning ahead for years to have money for my future. If I had waited until I retired, it would be too late to set aside enough money to help have a more comfortable retirement. I try to plan ahead for my health by exercising, attempting to eat right most of the time, and diligently managing my hypertension. It has been more difficult to plan ahead by creating the skills I will need for retirement because it seems I've learned well how to work but not how to not work. But this is something I can begin to practice by planning more time now for pleasurable activities and also for trying new things.

I am also planning for my memory to be less efficient than it is now. I have already begun to use more external memory aids and plan to continue to add to my storehouse. I have drawn up a Durable Power of Attorney, and I have a Living Will. I don't want to be reactive to aging but rather proactive on as many fronts as I can. I want to both enjoy and remember the rest of my life.

I have worked with many who have aged successfully. I have worked with many who have successfully planned ahead and managed significant memory loss in themselves or in someone for whom they care. Having memory loss does not have to lead to a loss of joy in life. Aging is not a disease that I must defeat. Successful aging is not aging without managing disease. Rather, to age successfully, I have to spend time now considering what is really important to me. I suspect that I will revise my plans several more times before my life is over.

Time and recollection are my most valued gifts. If I plan well the things that are important to me, I can use my time in the future to meet the goal set by Carl Rogers, a famous psychologist: Rather than growing older, I plan on being older and growing.

References and Bibliography

General Books and Chapters on Memory and Related Topics

Albert, M. S., & Moss, M. B. (Eds.). (1988). *Geriatric neuropsychology*. New York: Guilford.

Arden, J. B. (2002). *Improving your memory for dummies*. New York: Wiley.

Baddeley, A. (1986). *Working memory*. New York: Wiley.

Charness, N., & Bosman, E. A. (1992). Human factors and age. In F. I. M. Craik & T. A. Salthouse (Eds.) *The handbook of aging and cognition* (pp. 495–551). Hillsdale: Lawrence Earlbaum Associates.

Dudai, Y. (1989). *The neurobiology of memory: Concepts, findings, trends*. New York: Oxford.

Fisk, A. D., & Rogers, W. A. (Eds.). (1997). *Handbook of human factors and the older adult*. San Diego: Academic Press.

Gardner, H. (1974). *The shattered mind*. New York: Vintage.

Gordon, B. (1995). *Remembering and forgetting in everyday life*. New York: Mastermedia Limited.

Herrmann, D. J. (1990). *Super memory*. London: Blanford.

Herrmann, D. J., Weingartner, H., Searleman, A., & McEvoy, C. (Eds.). (1992). *Memory improvement: Implications for memory theory*. New York: Springer-Verlag.

Joyce, J. (1916). *A portrait of the artist as a young man*. New York: Signet.

La Rue, A. (1992). *Aging and neuropsychological assessment*. New York: Plenum.

Mason, D. J., & Kohn, M. L. (2001). *The memory workbook: Breakthrough techniques to exercise your brain and improve your memory*. Oakland: New Harbinger.

Neisser, U. (1976). *Cognition and reality: Principles and implications of cognitive psychology*. San Francisco: W. H. Freeman.

Park, D. C. (1992). Applied cognitive aging research. In F. I. M. Craik & T. A. Salthouse (Eds.) *The handbook of aging and cognition* (pp. 449–93). Hillsdale: Lawrence Earlbaum Associates.

Schacter, D. L. (Ed.). (1995). *Memory distortion: How minds, brains, and societies reconstruct the past*. Cambridge: Harvard University Press.

Schacter, D. L. (1996). *Searching for memory*. New York: Basic Books.

Schacter, D. L. (2001). *The seven sins of memory: How the mind forgets and remembers*. New York: Houghton Mifflin.

Small, G. (2002). *The memory bible*. New York: Hyperion.

Squire, L. R. (1987). *Memory and brain*. New York: Oxford.

Twain, M. (1995). How to make history dates stick. In S. Miller (Ed.), *Essays and sketches of Mark Twain* (pp. 215–22). New York: Barnes & Noble.

Twain, M. (1995). Taming the bicycle. In S. Miller (Ed.), *Essays and sketches of Mark Twain* (pp. 223–39). New York: Barnes & Noble.

Wilson, B. A., & Moffat, N. (Eds.). (1992). *Clinical management of memory problems*, second Edition. San Diego: Singular.

Wilson, B. A. (1987). *Rehabilitation of memory*. New York: Guilford Press.

Wingfield, A., & Byrnes, D. L. (1981). *The psychology of human memory*. New York: Academic Press.

Books on the Power of Personal Stories

Birren, J. E., & Feldman, L. (1997). *Where to go from here: Discovering your own life's wisdom in the second half of your life*. New York: Simon & Schuster.

Cohen, G. D. (2000). *The creative age: Awakening human potential in the second half of life*. New York: Avon Books.

Taylor, D. (1996). *The healing power of stories*. New York: Doubleday.

Your story: A guided interview through your personal and family history. Seattle: Seattle Aero, Inc.

General Books on Alzheimer's Disease and Caregiving

Castleman, M., Gallagher-Thompson, D., & Naythons, M. (1999). *There's still a person in there*. New York: Perigee.

Feil, N. (2002). *The validation breakthrough*, second edition. Baltimore: Health Professional Press.

Gray-Davidson, F. (1999). *The Alzheimer's sourcebook for caregivers*. Los Angeles: Lowell House.

Kuhn, D. (1999). *Alzheimer's early stages*. Alameda: Hunter House.

Mace, N. L., & Rabins, P. V. (1991). *The 36-hour day*, revised edition. Baltimore: Johns Hopkins University Press.

Peterson, R. (Ed.). (2002). *Mayo Clinic on Alzheimer's disease*. Rochester: Mayo Clinic Health Information.

Post, S. G. (2000). *The moral challenge of Alzheimer's disease*, second edition. Baltimore: Johns Hopkins University Press.

Shenk, D. (2001). *The forgetting. Alzheimer's: A portrait of an epidemic*. New York: Doubleday.

Warner, M. L. (1998). *The complete guide to Alzheimer's-proofing your home*. West Lafayette, Ind.: Purdue University Press.

Technical Books on Alzheimer's Disease and Caregiving

Albert, M. L., & Knoefel, J. E. (Eds.). (1994). *Clinical neurology of aging, second edition*. New York: Oxford.

Iqbal, K., Sisodia, S. S., & Winblad, B. (2001). *Alzheimer's disease: Advances in etiology, pathogenesis and therapeutics*. New York: Wiley.

Lichtenberg, P. A., Murman, D. L., & Mellow, A. M. (Eds.). (2003). *Handbook of dementia*. New York: Wiley.

Light, E., Niederhe, G., & Lebowitz, B. D., (Eds.). (1994). *Stress effects on family caregivers of Alzheimer's patients*. New York: Springer Publishing Company.

Morris, R. G. (Ed). (1996). *The cognitive neuropsychology of Alzheimer-type dementia*. New York: Oxford.

Mulligan, R., Van der Linden, M., & Juillerat, A-C. (Eds.). (2003). *The clinical management of early Alzheimer's disease*. Mahwah, N.J.: Lawrence Earlbaum Associates.

Parks, R. W., Zec, R. F., & Wilson, R. S. (1993). *Neuropsychology of Alzheimer's disease and other dementias*. New York: Oxford.

Whitehouse, P. J. (1993). *Dementia*, second edition. Philadelphia: F. A. Davis.

Books on Stress and Emotions

Antonovsky, A. (1979). *Health, stress, and coping*. San Francisco: Jossy-Bass.

Antonovsky, A. (1988). *Unraveling the mystery of health: How many people manage stress and stay well*. San Francisco: Jossy-Bass.

Barlow, D. H. (1988). *Anxiety and its disorders: The nature and treatment of anxiety and panic*. New York: Guilford.

Beck, A. T. (1967). *Depression: Clinical, experimental, and theoretical aspects*. New York: Hoeber.

Beck, A. T., Rush, A. J., Shaw, B. R., & Emery, G. (1979). *Cognitive therapy of depression*. New York: Guilford.

Beckham, E. E., & Leber, W. R. (Eds.). (1995). *Handbook of depression*, second edition. New York: Guilford.

Blazer, D. (2002). *Depression in late life*, second edition. New York: Springer.

Duffy, M. (Ed.). (1999). *Handbook of counseling and psychotherapy with older adults.* New York: Wiley.

D'Zurilla, T. M., & Nezu, A. M. (1999). *Problem-solving therapy: A social competence approach to clinical intervention,* second edition. New York: Springer.

Everly, Jr., G. S., & Lating, J. M. (2002). *A clinical guide to the treatment of the human stress response,* second edition. New York: Kluwer Academic/Plenum.

Lazarus, J. (2000). *Stress Relief & Relaxation Techniques.* Lincolnwood, Ill.: Keats.

Meichenbaum, D. (1985). *Stress inoculation training.* Oxford: Pergamon.

Miller, L. H., & Smith, A. D. (1993). *The stress solution: An action plan to manage stress in your life.* New York: Pocket Books.

Smith, J. C. (2002). *Stress management: A comprehensive handbook of techniques and strategies.* New York: Springer.

Journal Articles

Banks, W. A., & Morley, J. E. (2003). Memories are made of this: Recent advances in understanding cognitive impairments and dementia. *Journal of Gerontology: Medical Sciences, 58A,* 314–21.

Blazer, D. G. (2003). Depression in late life: Review and commentary. *Journal of Gerontology: Medical Sciences, 58A,* 249–65.

Brown, S. C., & Park, D. C. (2003). Theoretical models of cognitive aging and implications for translational research in medicine. *The Gerontologist, 43,* Special Issue, 57–67.

DeKosky, S. T. (2003). Pathology and pathways of Alzheimer's disease with an update on new developments in treatment. *Journal of the American Geriatrics Society, 5* (Supplement), S314–20.

Fillit, H. M., et al. (2002). Achieving and maintaining cognitive vitality with aging. *Mayo Clinic Proceedings, 77,* 681–96.

Geldmacher, D. S. (2003). Alzheimer's disease: Current pharmacotherapy in the context of patient and family needs. *Journal of the American Geriatrics Society, 5* (Supplement), S289–95.

Gitlin, L. N., Liebman, J., & Winter, L. (2003). Are environmental interventions effective in the management of Alzheimer's disease and related disorders? *Alzheimer's Care Quarterly, 4,* 85–107.

Grossberg, G. T., & Desai, A. K. (2003). Management of Alzheimer's disease. *Journal of Gerontology: Medical Sciences, 58A,* 331–53.

Haak, N. J. (2002). Maintaining connections: Understanding communication from the perspective of persons with dementia. *Alzheimer's Care Quarterly, 2,* 116–131.

Haak, N. J. (2003). "Do you hear what I mean?" A lived experience of disrupted communication in mid-to-late state Alzheimer's disease. *Alzheimer's Care Quarterly, 4,* 26–40.

Kirshner, H. S. (2003). Medical prevention of stroke, *Southern Medical Journal, 96,* 354–58.

Leifer. B. P. (2003). Early diagnosis of Alzheimer's disease: Clinical and economic benefits. *Journal of the American Geriatrics Society, 5* (Supplement), S281–88.

Mehta, K. M., et al. (2003). Additive effects of cognitive function and depressive symptoms on mortality in elderly community-living adults. *Journal of Gerontology: Medical Sciences, 58A,* 461–67.

Roman, G. C. (2003). Vascular dementia: Distinguishing characteristics, treatment, and prevention. *Journal of the American Geriatrics Society, 5* (Supplement), S296–S304.

Strub, R. (2003). Vascular dementia. *Southern Medical Journal, 96,* 363–66.

Truscott, M. (2003). Life in the slow lane. *Alzheimer's Care Quarterly, 4,* 11–17.

Zakzanis, K. K., Graham, S. J., & Campbell, Z. (2003). A metanalysis of structural and functional brain imaging in dementia. *Neuropsychology Review, 13,* 1–18.

About the Author

For more than 30 years, **DR. BILL BECKWITH** has been studying, researching, and teaching about memory. He has earned advanced degrees in Experimental Psychology and Clinical Psychology from The Ohio State University.

His extensive career as an educator spans decades of teaching—from preschool to graduate students. As a Professor at the University of North Dakota, Dr. Beckwith

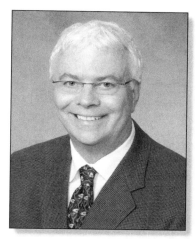

BILL E. BECKWITH, Ph.D.

was honored with several teaching awards and grants. As a researcher, Dr. Beckwith has broadened our knowledge of neuroscience, learning, and memory. He has been published extensively in these fields.

During the past decade, Dr. Beckwith has focused on the needs of people with memory loss and their caregivers by developing important new approaches and programs. He led and trained others as the clinical director of a major memory disorders clinic. He also established the Department of Behavioral Health and created the innovative Center for Excellence in Memory Care for a large retirement community.

Aware of the increasing interest in and need for practical knowledge about memory, this renowned educator now brings his expertise to broader audiences. Dr. Beckwith and his wife, Pamela, are founders of Memory Management. This educational resource company is dedicated to aiding people in planning and managing their memory assets through seminars, workshops, publications, and consultations.

Additional information about Dr. Beckwith and Memory Management, as well as up-to-date contact information, can be found on the Internet at www.memorymanagement.info.

Index